MW00849992

For Oona Fessenden and A.N.V. Rao, devoted teachers.

The
CRISPR
Generation

The Story of the World's First
Gene-Edited Babies

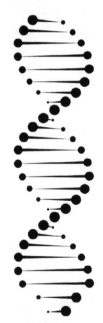

Kiran Musunuru

Copyright 2019

All rights reserved. This book or any portion thereof may not be reproduced or used in any manner whatsoever without the express written permission of the publisher except for the use of brief quotations in a book review.

ISBN 978-1-54398-637-2 (print)
ISBN 978-1-54398-638-9 (eBook)

Contents

Prologue

The auditorium was filled to capacity. Hundreds of people from across the globe had come to Hong Kong to attend the Second International Summit on Human Genome Editing. They were now waiting for the main event of the three-day conference. The event no one had planned for.

It was standing room only, which was not unheard of for a scientific talk of broad interest. Most unusually, however, the main aisle was packed with reporters, many with large cameras at the ready. Security personnel prowled in front of the stage. Though the audience was hushed, the room was electric with anticipation. More than a million people around the world watched a livestream of the proceedings. History was about to be unveiled. Whether it was a historic scientific achievement or a historic ethical fiasco would soon be known.

Two days earlier, Dr. He Jiankui had announced via YouTube that his team had produced the world's first gene-edited babies. The twins Lulu and Nana—the first citizens of the CRISPR generation. To the vast majority of people in the room, it came as a shock, a slap in the face. The very reason for the Summit in the first place was concern that the ability to edit the genes of babies was within reach. The goal was to ensure that it was not done prematurely, and if it was going to be done someday, that it be done transparently, ethically, and safely. Now it appeared that Dr. He had gone rogue and just done it anyway. The general feeling was that the way in which he had done it was neither transparent, nor ethical, nor safe. But nobody could be sure about this, because the details of Dr. He's project were still under wraps. Many suspected that his claim of gene-edited babies was an elaborate hoax.

Now Dr. He would be giving his first scientific presentation since making his announcement. The world would finally see what he had been up to. He would face his peers and his many detractors for the first time.

The moderator gave a short introduction, stressing to the audience the principles of free speech and respect. He asked Dr. He to come to the stage and present his work. He then looked around uttering, "I don't know where he is …"

Ten seconds passed, then twenty seconds, then thirty seconds. People looked around, but Dr. He was not in the auditorium. Was he at the conference? Was he even in Hong Kong? The world waited with bated breath to see if Dr. He would dare to show up and defend himself.

At that moment, only a handful of people knew the truth about Lulu and Nana, the full story of how they'd come to be, the terrible act that had been committed in the name of the greater good. I was one of them.

1

THE RNA WORLD

To understand CRISPR, you need to understand the RNA world.

Genetics is fundamentally about the molecule called deoxyribonu-cleic acid, or DNA. Nowadays, biologists and physicians—and, increasingly, members of the lay public—obsess about the information content of DNA molecules in the body. DNA is rather boring, though, compared to the molecule called ribonucleic acid, or RNA.

As any researcher who works on RNA will tell you, we actually live in an RNA world. Life on earth is believed to have arisen specifically because of RNA—it is an amazingly flexible and versatile molecule. It is made up of four different building blocks, or bases: adenine, abbreviated as A; cytosine, or C; guanine, or G; and uracil, or U. The RNA molecule itself is an assembly of bases into a sequence in a single strand (Figure 1). Essentially, there is an infinite number of possible combinations of the four bases that could make up RNA strands. Imagine a typewriter with four keys. Start hitting those keys in a random order, and type a word of any length. That is one potential RNA base sequence. Do it again, and you have another potential RNA base sequence.

DIFFERENCES
BETWEEN DNA & RNA

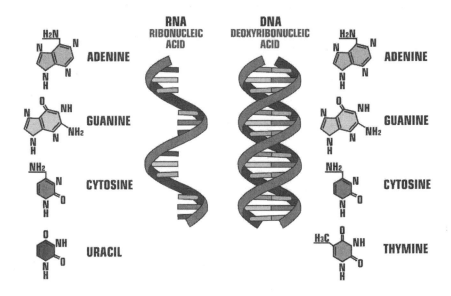

FIGURE 1

What does it mean to be in an RNA world? In early life, billions of years ago, RNA played a number of roles. Certain RNA strands with the right sequences folded up on themselves in interesting ways, used their contours to grab onto other molecules, and facilitated chemical changes to those molecules. In scientific parlance, we consider these RNA strands to be enzymes. Some RNA strands turned their enzymatic activity on themselves, cleaving themselves into shorter strands, each of which might go on to fulfill its own unique role. Yet other RNA strands used their bases as a repository of information. They engaged with other molecules—

some RNA, some not—that read out the base sequences and used them to build a different type of molecule, proteins. Those proteins then went on to do other important things. Because the base sequences wouldn't themselves be changed during the process of making proteins, the RNA strands could be read out—translated—over and over again to produce lots of protein molecules.

Most crucially, RNA could reproduce itself. This takes advantage of an unusual symmetry among the RNA bases. Each base has the ability to pair off with another base: adenine with uracil, cytosine with guanine, guanine with cytosine, uracil with adenine. This ability is inherent in the chemical structures of the bases. Consider an RNA strand with the sequence ACUG. It can be faithfully copied through an elaborate procedure. A separate second strand of RNA is constructed from bases that paired with the first strand's sequence. For the A in the first position in the original strand, the second strand incorporates a U, since A and U pair off. For the C in the second position, the second strand incorporates a G. For the U in the third position, an A. For the G in the fourth position, a C. So the second strand is U+G+A+C.

Now the original RNA molecule moves off. The second strand can now serve as a template in its own right to produce a third strand. In the first position of the third strand, it incorporates an A to match up with the U in the second strand. The second, third, and fourth positions of the third strand: C, U, and finally G. This third strand is identical to the first strand. Mission accomplished! The second strand continues to serve as a template for the production of more copies of the original strand, or it can simply be broken down and discarded. The new copies of the original RNA strand can then serve to fortify existing life, or perhaps go forth to seed new life.

In the dance of molecules that gave form to early life, RNA reigned supreme. But its wondrous dynamism comes at a steep cost. RNA is highly vulnerable to its environment. If something occurs to cause a change in any of the bases in the RNA sequence—for example, a chemical conversion of a cytosine base to a uracil base—there is no way for the RNA molecule to recover from that change. If the original sequence read ACUG, it now reads AUUG. This change is what we call a mutation, and there is no way to repair it. It might result in a permanent change in the RNA's function, or perhaps in a change of the function of an altered protein built from the readout of the altered RNA sequence. In an even more dire scenario, chemicals in the environment can act to break down the RNA molecule altogether, degrading it beyond any possibility of recovery. Whatever function or information was in that RNA is now lost forever. Life that formed around RNA as its central molecule was precarious.

In the RNA world, at some point in the history of earthly life, some life-forms developed a trick that gave them a tremendous advantage over other life-forms. During the copying of RNA and creation of a second strand from the original strand, the two strands stuck together permanently in a double-strand structure. Chemical changes over time served to stabilize this structure. The bases that paired off between the first and second strands were perpetually locked into place as so-called base pairs, and each uracil was replaced with the chemically similar thymine, or T, which, like uracil, readily forms base pairs with adenine. This is how the first DNA molecules were born. The two strands of DNA wind around each other in an extremely stable double-helix configuration. The base pairs lie in the core of the double helix, protected from the environment (Figure 1). The information in the DNA base pair sequence was far more secure than it had ever been in the RNA form.

Changes to individual bases still occurred in DNA, but much less readily and less frequently. And because each base was paired up with a base in the other strand, it made for a buddy system of sorts. There was now a way to repair accidental base changes—remove the base and replace it with a fresh base matching up with the base in the other strand. If a base pair across the two strands was originally A–T, and something happened to change the A on the first strand into a G—a chance encounter with a toxin, or radiation from the sun—the G on the first strand and the T on the second strand would no longer be properly paired. One of two things would then occur. First, the G on the first strand could be removed and replaced with an A to pair with the T on the second strand, repairing the A-to-G base change and restoring the original sequence. Second, the T could be removed from the second strand and replaced with a C to pair with the G on the first strand, resulting in a permanent change of the original A–T base pair into a G–C base pair: a mutation. There are roughly equal odds of successful repair of the base change versus a mutation. Not perfect, but a big improvement on the situation with RNA.

The life-forms that developed DNA had a substantial advantage over the life-forms with RNA only—so much so that they ended up taking over all earthly life. We and all other existing organisms are their descendants. Billions of years ago, all life was still in the form of individual cells, each living or dying according to its own circumstances. Those cells blessed with the stability of the DNA molecule thrived and multiplied. As the full advantages of DNA became manifest, the cells evolved, packing more and more information into each DNA molecule until it contained all of the information necessary to produce and direct all of the cell's molecular machinery. DNA had become the repository of the blueprint of life.

Each cell copied its DNA molecule similarly to the copying of RNA. In a process called replication, the two DNA strands served as templates to build two new strands. The four strands coalesced into two identical double-helix DNA molecules. When a cell divided, it passed a DNA copy to each of its two daughter cells. DNA became the mechanism of inheritance, passing along genetic information from generation to generation. Even after cells assembled into multicellular life-forms and evolved into complex organisms such as humans, DNA continues to serve that same purpose.

Yet the advantages of DNA come at a cost. DNA is stable, dependable, and committed to its purpose for the long haul. But it is boring. It can't do much besides serving as a lockbox to safeguard the genetic information. It lacks the versatility of RNA. So, life evolved to repurpose RNA as a short-lived instrument to convey the instructions contained in DNA. In scientific parlance, base pair sequences in DNA are organized as discrete units called genes, and these sequences are transcribed into RNA base sequences. A collection of proteins (called the transcription machinery) unwinds two DNA strands at the site of a gene, and uses one of the strands as a template to construct an RNA molecule. The RNA strand's sequence perfectly matches the gene sequence in the DNA, except that U substitutes for T. The RNA is mobile, and with some modifications becomes so-called messenger RNA. The messenger RNA travels away from the DNA from which it was transcribed to another part of the cell. There the messenger RNA encounters a large molecular machine—built from RNAs and proteins—called the ribosome, which reads out the RNA base sequence and translates it into building blocks—amino acids—that are assembled into a fresh new protein.

This process is known as the central dogma: the genetic information flows from DNA to RNA, via transcription, and from RNA to protein, via translation. The central dogma governs our lives at a scale far too microscopic for us to perceive in our everyday lives. Except when errors in the information content of the DNA base pair sequence—mutations—propagate through RNAs, proteins, cells, organs, and the body, causing disease and suffering.

The central dogma holds that genetic information flows in one direction only, away from DNA. There is no way for new information to be encoded deliberately into DNA. DNA is a lockbox.

Some of the earliest forms of earthly life, single-cell microbes we know as bacteria, found themselves vulnerable to parasites we know as viruses. Some types of viruses were devilishly simple, little more than a DNA molecule wrapped in a protein coating. They lacked the elaborate machinery normally associated with life. Each virus was entirely inert, dead to the world, until it came into contact with the right type of bacterium. Then the virus used its protein coating to invade the bacterium, to smuggle its DNA molecule into the interior of the bacterial cell.

The virus hijacked the bacterium's replication, transcription, and translation machinery. The viral DNA molecule proliferated into many copies sharing the same sequence. In keeping with the central dogma, the genetic information in the viral DNA passed via transcription into RNA molecules and then via translation into proteins. Some of these proteins assembled into new coatings to wrap around the copied viral DNA molecules, and other proteins aided in the assembly process. From a single virus infecting a single bacterium, many new viruses burst out into the world, killing the hapless bacterium. The host of new viruses had the potential to victimize many more bacteria as fodder for their own reproduction.

In response to the onslaught of viruses, bacteria evolved a variety of countermeasures. The most sophisticated of these defenses represented a violation of the central dogma. Some bacteria figured out how to slice and dice viral DNA molecules and incorporate the small pieces into their own DNA molecules. These bacteria could open the lockbox and add new information, a recording of viral signatures that would then be passed on from generation to generation of bacteria. In and of itself, this historical record of past encounters with viruses wouldn't do much good. DNA couldn't do anything more than serve as an archive. So the bacteria created molecular machines that exploited the new information in their DNA. These machines were sentinels that could crisscross the bacterial cell and detect any foreign DNA molecules—including any DNA from an invading virus. As with many other molecular machines in the cell, these sentinels had both protein and RNA components.

What made these sentinels uniquely powerful was that they contained RNA molecules transcribed from the archive of viral signatures in the bacterial DNA. These RNA molecules, of course, had the same genetic information as the information in the archive. Not only did the sentinels detect foreign DNA molecules, they quickly scanned the entirety of the foreign DNAs and looked for matches with the viral signatures. If there was a perfect match between any single viral signature in RNA and some part of the sequence of the foreign DNA, it would mean that the bacterium (or one of its ancestors) had survived an encounter with that kind of virus in the past. The sentinel would then cut the foreign DNA into pieces and forestall the construction of new viruses, saving the bacterium from an untimely death. In other words, the sentinels were built to search and destroy, in a primitive version of the immune systems that would later evolve in complex multicellular organisms like animals.

Eons later, a species called *Homo sapiens* would intensively study these bacteria and discover these archives and sentinels, giving them the catchall name of CRISPR. And human beings would figure out how to reverse-engineer CRISPR and use it to violate the central dogma, to open the lockbox, to rewrite their own DNA—and, maybe, to take control of their own evolution.

2

THE MAN WITH A THOUSAND HOLES IN HIS BRAIN

We are all mutants.

You might be in pristine health. Maybe you have never been in a hospital except to visit a sick family member or friend. Maybe you have never had anything worse than the common cold. You are still a mutant.

Like every other human being on earth, your body bears dozens of mutations—changes in your genetic information—that are unique to you—or shared only with some of your children and grandchildren, if you have any. Perhaps you are lucky and none of your mutations have any meaning for your health. Or you are unlucky and one of your mutations has profound consequences, and you suffer from a serious disease that runs in your family.

Perhaps you're healthy enough that you think you're one of the lucky ones, but in fact a mutation might be causing all sorts of mischief in your body without you knowing it. The resilience of the human body, its ability to accommodate genetic mistakes, is incredible.

I learned just how incredible when I met the man with a thousand holes in his brain.

I did my graduate studies at The Rockefeller University in New York City as part of a joint MD–PhD program in which I trained as a scientist and as a physician, the latter at Cornell University Medical College across the street. Rockefeller has a rich history when it comes to DNA. It is the place where Drs. Oswald Avery, Colin MacLeod, and Maclyn McCarty famously discovered in the 1940s that DNA, not RNA or protein, is the repository of genetic information. During the ensuing decades, Rockefeller hosted a variety of researchers who made seminal discoveries related to DNA and the processes of replication and transcription. Yet by the time I started my studies at Rockefeller in the late 1990s, the study of RNA was coming into its own. Researchers were starting to appreciate the versatility of RNA molecules and to flesh out the details of prehistoric life in the RNA world. I was captivated by the new science, and my graduate studies ended up becoming an extended fling with RNA. I gave barely any thought to DNA, genetics, and how mutations cause disease.

My first real exposure to genetics was through an elective medical training experience during my last year in graduate school at Rockefeller. I had finished two years of medical school before starting graduate school, and I would be going back to complete the last two years of medical school after defending my PhD thesis. The final years would be a gauntlet of intense, sleep-deprived rotations across the whole gamut of medical specialties. So I wanted to spend some time getting reacquainted with the medical side of things while wrapping up my graduate studies. I'd spent the last few years in a laboratory studying RNA molecules involved in diseases of the brain, yet I hadn't had much experience taking care of actual patients with these diseases. In early 2003, I arranged to spend several weeks working with Dr. Raj Murali, a senior neurosurgeon at the now-defunct St. Vincent's Hospital in Manhattan. I observed many surgical cases involving the brain and spinal cord and helped take care of patients before and after the surgeries. It marked the first time I ever saw a living human brain with my own eyes—quite a sight to see.

About midway through my time with Murali, he introduced me to a patient who would soon be undergoing surgery on the spinal cord. The patient was an affable African-American man, sixty years of age, who had been in good health all his life, with no problems until four years earlier. He started to feel tingling in the fingers of his right hand. He eventually was diagnosed with carpal tunnel syndrome and treated for it. This seemed to fix the problem, but two months earlier he'd suffered a recurrence of the symptoms in his right hand, and this time they included numbness and weakness as well. He was fairly stoic about the symptoms. Left to his own devices, he would have just gone on uncomplainingly with his life. But his wife noticed that he was having trouble buttoning his shirt and had switched to his left hand to get the task done. She persuaded him to have his symptoms checked by a physician.

The neurologist who evaluated him arranged for an MRI scan to look for any problems in the spinal cord. Lo and behold, there was a large mass pressing on his spinal cord at the level of his neck. This perfectly explained his symptoms. One of the nerves running through that part of the spinal cord ran through the arm into the right hand and carried signals back and forth from the fingers. By squeezing on that nerve bundle within the spinal cord, the mass caused problems in the hand itself.

The next step was obvious. The neurologist consulted Murali about an operation to remove the mass and relieve the pressure on the spinal cord. With any luck, the patient would recover the full use of his hand. But there was a wrinkle. When the two physicians looked over the results of the MRI scan, they saw more than one mass in the spinal cord. There were two additional, smaller masses, one at the level of the lower neck and one at the level of the upper back. Neither looked to be causing any problems, but there was no good explanation why there were multiple masses. Because problems that affect the spinal cord can also affect the brain, the patient underwent an additional MRI scan, this one of the entire brain.

Murali showed me the results of the brain scan. It was astounding. It looked like there were gaping holes—lesions, in medical parlance— throughout the brain (Figure 2). The largest was perhaps the size of a walnut, but the lesions varied greatly in size, including some of pinpoint size on the scan. This meant that there were lots of tinier lesions that could not be picked up by the MRI scan. There were easily a thousand or more of these lesions in this man's head, which was difficult to square with his absolutely normal appearance and demeanor when I met him. How could he be doing so well with a brain so riddled with holes?

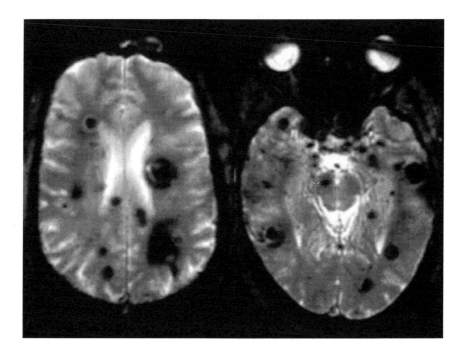

FIGURE 2

Seeing my confusion, Murali explained what was going on. These lesions were not holes but rather areas of blood, which showed up as black on the images. Each of these lesions was a so-called cavernoma, a cluster of abnormal blood vessels with bubbles of blood that to the naked eye would look like mulberries, dark red to purple in color. Another name for the phenomenon was cerebral cavernous malformation (CCM). Cavernomas are slow-growing, with a time course of years, which meant that the brain tissue surrounding around each lesion had time to accommodate to the growing mass. It was a testament to the wondrous resilience of the human body that the patient had no idea what was going on inside his skull, perceiving himself to be in perfect health. But the spinal cord is confined to a narrow space within the bones of the spine that one can feel along the back. There is less ability for tissue in the spinal cord to adjust to a growing mass, which is why the patient's first serious problem was related to a mass in the spinal cord, not one in the brain.

Perhaps one in two hundred people have a single cavernoma in the brain, and most never realize it and never have problems from it. But there was clearly something very unusual going on with this patient—he didn't have just one, or ten, or one hundred cavernomas. He clearly had an unusual predisposition to form these cavernomas. That could mean only one thing, I thought: a genetic issue. Something lurking in his DNA, an error in one of the gene sequences, was at fault. I asked Murali what was known about the genetics of CCM. Not much, he said, although it was known to run in families, especially in Hispanic families in the Southwestern United States.

I wanted to know more, so in my spare time I went to the library to do some reading. It turned out that, coincidently, just a few years earlier, a group of researchers in France and a group of researchers in the United States had each discovered that a gene called *KRIT1* was responsible for familial CCM. (For reference, gene names are always in italics, and protein names are not.) *KRIT1* did not explain all cases of familial CCM; later, two additional genes would be linked to the condition. But at the time, *KRIT1* was the only clue I had as to a possible explanation for the man with a thousand lesions.

I was in the operating room when Murali performed surgery on the patient. It went smoothly, without any complications. When Murali opened up the delicate layer lining the spinal cord within the bones of the spine, it revealed the mass. It did, indeed, look like a small cluster of fruit. Murali carefully dissected the cavernoma away from the spinal cord and removed it, relieving the pressure on the spinal cord. The job complete, he closed up the spine and sent the patient to the recovery room.

As the patient was convalescing in the hospital, I told Murali about what I had learned from my reading. Perhaps we should see if the patient has a mutation in his *KRIT1* gene, I suggested. Murali was not experienced with genetics but encouraged me to investigate further. I came back with a proposal—let's get a blood sample from the patient and use the DNA in that sample to determine the base pair sequence in his *KRIT1* gene. We can check to see if there is any deviation from the normal sequence, a mutation, that could explain his thousand lesions. Murali enthusiastically supported this proposal, and we spoke to the head of the hospital's Institutional Review Board, the ethics committee responsible for overseeing any research involving patients in the hospital.

After obtaining approval to proceed, we sat down with the patient just before he was ready to go home. We explained that we wished to see if we could identify a gene mutation responsible for his condition, and then went through the benefits and risks of the procedure. The major benefits: we might be able to give him an explanation for his disease, and the study could add to our knowledge about familial CCM and potentially help other patients with the disease. The risks were simply those associated with any routine blood draw, which are quite minor—a brief bit of pain, a little bleeding. After we answered his questions about the procedure, the patient consented to the study.

We also asked the patient more about his medical history. Did he remember ever having any problems with his brain? During previous conversations, he hadn't recalled any issues, but now he told us something new: he'd had a couple of seizures in the past. When asked whether any of his family members had a similar problem—he had previously reported that they'd all been healthy—he said, oh sure, my sister had a lot of seizures when she was still alive and took medication for them. Was it possible that the patient and his sister shared a *KRIT1* mutation that caused both to have cavernomas in the brain that resulted in seizures?

We would never know for sure about his sister, since she was deceased. But with a blood sample from the patient, we could at least figure out his situation. Because I was a graduate student working in a state-of-the-art laboratory at Rockefeller, I had at my disposal the necessary tools to analyze the patient's DNA. I started by processing the tube of blood and isolating the cells. There are several types of cells in human blood, including red blood cells, white blood cells, and platelets. Of these, only white blood cells have appreciable amounts of DNA. Treatment of these cells with certain chemicals released the DNA, which I was then able to purify using other chemicals.

Now came the tricky part. The DNA that I now had in a test tube contained the entirety of the DNA base pair sequences present in the patient's cells. Each human cell has a collection of forty-six large DNA molecules, known as chromosomes, contained within a central compartment of the cell, the nucleus. The genetic information is spread out all across the forty-six chromosomes—a total of about 6.4 billion base pairs of DNA sequence—which together make up the human genome. These chromosomes are actually twenty-three pairs of chromosomes. These chromosomes are numbered 1 through 22, ordered by decreasing size (chromosome 1 is the largest). The twenty-third chromosome pair determines whether a person is biologically a woman or a man and comes in two versions—a larger X chromosome and a smaller Y chromosome that have different genes. With some exceptions, women have two X chromosomes in each cell, and men have one X and one Y chromosome.

The chromosomes within each pair are largely identical (with the exception of the X and Y chromosomes), but do have occasional mismatches in the DNA base pair sequence all along the length of the strands. These mismatches, also called variants, are what make each person unique. One of the chromosomes in each pair is inherited from the person's mother, the other chromosome from the father. The variants that come from the mother are what make a person similar to the mother in all sorts of characteristics such as appearance, health, and risk of disease. Likewise, the variants inherited from the father make for similarity to the father. Having a mix of variants from the mother and father makes the person a true hybrid of the parents. Because of the pairing of chromosomes in this fashion, most genes in the genome are present in two versions—two copies—one from the mother and one from the father.

I had my patient's full genetic information in a tube of DNA. But I didn't care about all 6.4 billion base pairs in the human genome. I really only wanted to know what was in the *KRIT1* gene, which is located in one spot on chromosome 7. The sequence of interest was just 2,200 base pairs in length—times two, to cover both copies of the gene on the chromosome 7 pair. Determining just this tiny amount of sequence from the entire genome was like picking a needle out of a very large haystack. Fortunately, since it was 2003, I was poised to take advantage of the fruits of three technological revolutions: one from the 1980s, one from the 1990s, and one from the early 2000s.

The most recent of the advances was the Human Genome Project. An international effort spearheaded by the U.S. National Institutes of Health and the U.S. Department of Energy, its goals were to determine the full DNA base pair sequences across the twenty-three chromosome pairs and to precisely identify and map the locations of all of the genes. Launched in 1990, it was declared complete in 2003 at a cost of about $3 billion, having identified about twenty thousand protein-coding genes in the human genome.

Although the timing might have seemed ideal for the work I wanted to do, the data from the Human Genome Project were not yet organized and accessible in the way I needed. (Though I and innumerable other researchers have tremendously benefited from the data in the years since.)

Instead, I went to an alternative source. Dr. J. Craig Venter had founded the company Celera Genomics in 1998 with the goal of sequencing the human genome as a private effort paralleling the Human Genome Project. The initial business model was to sell access to Celera's proprietary sequence database to researchers willing to pay thousands of U.S. dollars in fees each year. At the time, Celera's competition with the federal government with an eye toward making a profit was controversial, but because the sequence data were so useful, my research mentor had signed up for Celera's service. Therefore I had the ability to trawl through Celera's data to find exactly what I needed—the sequence of the *KRIT1* gene.

I now needed a way to pick out and purify the patient's *KRIT1* sequence from the billions of base pairs in the genome. The technology that enabled me to do this was the polymerase chain reaction (PCR). PCR was implemented for the first time by Dr. Kary Mullis at Cetus Corporation in 1983, although the concept had been proposed twelve years earlier by Dr. H. Gobind Khorana at the University of Wisconsin–Madison. The work was of such monumental importance to biomedical research that Mullis was awarded the Nobel Prize in Chemistry in 1993. He would later come to be regarded as a colorful character with a penchant for supporting controversial views, such as denying that the HIV virus is the cause of AIDS and expressing a belief in astrology. But nobody questions the importance of his work with PCR.

PCR works like a molecular photocopier that can take a single copy of a DNA base pair sequence and churn out millions, billions, trillions of copies of that same sequence. This can be done in just a few hours with relatively inexpensive equipment and chemicals. Solving my problem of isolating the patient's *KRIT1* sequence didn't require me to physically separate out that sequence from the rest of the genome. I could simply use PCR to make a vast number of copies of the *KRIT1* sequence and leave the rest of the genome alone. By the time I was done, the amount of DNA with the *KRIT1* sequence in my final tube would so dwarf the rest of the DNA that it would be a near-pure preparation of my desired sequence.

To put it another way, if I had an auditorium full of people wanting to read a single page of a single very large book, I wouldn't bother to turn through all the pages of the book, find the right page, mark that page, and then have the book passed around for everybody to take turns reading. Instead, I would print out lots of copies of the page I needed and hand out those copies.

But PCR has an important limitation. In order for it to work, one needs to precisely define the boundaries of the DNA region to be amplified—point A to point B. All of the DNA base pair sequence between A and B is copied, and everything else is ignored. Crucially, one has to know the specific bases right at points A and B, because PCR requires the use of so-called primers that match those bases. Without knowing those bases, PCR is a non-starter.

That is why I needed access to the data from Celera. It provided me with the full DNA base pair sequence of the *KRIT1* gene and, just as important, the sequences surrounding the gene. I could make primers to set the boundaries at points just outside the gene and make sure to amplify the entirety of the gene sequence with PCR, rather than haphazardly amplifying some parts of the gene and missing other parts. I ended up designing sixteen sets of primers to kick-start sixteen PCR amplifications that would cover one hundred percent of the *KRIT1* gene sequence. This would guarantee that I did not miss the hoped-for mutation, which might be located anywhere in the gene sequence. It might even be at the very beginning or the very end of the gene.

The question now was whether the PCR amplifications would work. Despite one's most careful planning and best efforts, PCR can fail. The only way to know what would happen with PCR was to actually try it. I mixed the purified genomic DNA from the patient's blood with each of the sixteen primer sets and the necessary ingredients. I placed the sixteen tubes in the PCR machine and started it running. The process took a few hours to complete. At the end of that time, I analyzed the DNA in each of the tubes. I was hoping to see a large amount of DNA, meaning that the PCR had worked to make billions of copies. Beyond that, I wanted to see that the amplified DNA molecules were the correct length, consistent with the boundaries set by the primers in each tube. The moment of truth came … and I saw that all sixteen PCR amplifications had worked as hoped!

On to the last step. Now I had to use the PCR-amplified *KRIT1* gene sequence to read out the bases, one letter at a time, and see if I could find a mutation. I knew the normal *KRIT1* sequence from the Celera data. I was hoping to find a mismatch somewhere in the patient's *KRIT1* sequence. Now the third revolutionary technology came into play. I would use a technique known as Sanger sequencing, developed by Dr. Frederick Sanger in Cambridge, England, in 1977. (This technique won Sanger his second Nobel Prize in Chemistry, in 1980.) Sanger sequencing really took off in the 1990s when it was paired with a method called capillary electrophoresis that allowed for automation of the process. Automated Sanger sequencing has proven so useful in reading out the base pairs in DNA sequences that it's routinely used by laboratories to this day, costing just a few U.S. dollars per DNA sample. The output is a picture called a chromatogram. Scanning across a chromatogram from left to right, one sees a series of peaks. Each peak marks a single position in the DNA base pair sequence. The peaks are color-coded, with different colors for each of the four bases. Counting off the peaks in order and translating the colors into bases spells out the DNA sequence.

By 2003, Rockefeller had set up a facility where any researcher could submit DNA samples for automated Sanger sequencing. The facility could reliably read out several hundred base pairs of DNA sequence from each individual sample. The results were available electronically after just a couple of days. So all I had to do was submit my PCR-amplified DNA samples to the facility and wait to get the results back. By inspecting the sixteen chromatograms, I could assemble the entire sequence of the patient's *KRIT1* gene.

While I was waiting for the results, I thought carefully about what features I would expect to see in a chromatogram if the patient turned out to have a mutation in *KRIT1*. I would be looking through the chromatogram for evidence of a mutation in a single position in the DNA base pair sequence, a mismatch from the normal sequence. But there was a catch. Everyone has two versions of *KRIT1* in their genome, so the patient would as well, one on each of the chromosomes in the chromosome 7 pair. From my reading, I knew that patients with familial CCM typically had a mutation in only one version of *KRIT1*; the other version was normal. Having just one mutation was sufficient to cause full-blown disease. I had no reason to think that my patient would be any different.

Now, the crucial point: if PCR is used to amplify a gene sequence out of genomic DNA, it will actually amplify both versions of the gene simultaneously. This doesn't matter at all if both versions are normal; the PCR copies made from the two versions will be indistinguishable, since they will have exactly the same sequence. But if the two versions of the gene are mismatched, about half of the PCR copies will be amplified from the normal version, and the other half of the PCR copies from the mutant version. Put another way, if the PCR resulted in one hundred billion copies of the gene sequence in the tube, around fifty billion would be normal, and fifty billion would contain the mutation. If that PCR sample were submitted for automated Sanger sequencing, there wouldn't be a single well-defined peak at the position of the mutation in the chromatogram. Instead there would be two overlapping peaks, one with the color corresponding to the normal base in that position, and one with another color corresponding to the mismatched base in that position.

When I received the sixteen chromatograms, I knew what I was hoping to find: a position where there were two overlapping peaks of different colors. And on one of the chromatograms, I found exactly that!

But it wasn't enough to have simply found a mismatch, a mutation. I needed to understand whether the mutation had any real-world meaning. Mutations occur all the time, and almost all of them are benign, with no relevance to a person's health. It's possible the single mutation I had found in the *KRIT1* gene in my patient was benign, in which case I would be no closer to an answer than when I started. So I needed to understand the consequences of this particular mutation and determine whether it was the cause of the patient's disease.

The central dogma says that information proceeds from DNA to RNA to protein. The translation of a gene's base pair sequence into a protein is governed by the genetic code. Each consecutive group of three bases forms a so-called codon. Each codon represents an amino acid; a string of amino acids makes up a protein. There are sixty-four codons (considering all possible combinations of the four bases in each of the three positions in the codon: four x four x four). Sixty-one of the codons correspond to twenty amino acids. There's a lot of redundancy in this genetic code, with each amino acid coded by as few as one codon and as many as six codons. The first codon (start codon) of any gene is ATG, which is transcribed into AUG in the messenger RNA, which in turn is translated by the ribosome into the amino acid methionine.

When a ribosome encounters a messenger RNA, it scans along the base sequence until it sees a start codon. After incorporating a methionine, the ribosome then crawls along to the next codon (the next three RNA bases after AUG) and translates it into a second amino acid according to the genetic code. It adds that amino acid to the first methionine. The ribosome continues to crawl along, adding another amino acid for each codon it translates. It doesn't go on endlessly. Three of the codons—UAG, UGA, UAA—are stop codons. When the ribosome encounters a stop codon, it releases both the messenger RNA and the amino acid chain, which becomes a protein. Proteins have a variety of roles: structural components to build parts of the body, enzymes that foster chemical reactions on other molecules, signals that serve as communication between different cells or organs, and antibodies to fight off infections. After completing a protein, a ribosome can move on to start scanning another messenger RNA, and the process of protein building begins again.

When it comes to a gene sequence, there are several types of mutations that can occur. The first type is one we do not worry about much. Here, the mutation is confined to one position in the gene sequence. It changes a single codon, but does so in such a way that the new codon still codes for the same amino acid as the original codon. Despite the change in DNA (and messenger RNA) sequence, the protein will be exactly the same. It is very likely that this type of mutation will be silent and have no consequences at all.

The second type of mutation is also confined to one position in the gene sequence and changes a single codon. Here, the new codon codes for a different amino acid than the original codon. One amino acid in the protein will be changed. This might or might not affect the ability of the protein to carry out its normal function. To understand why, imagine copying a sentence from a book by typing it out. If one of the letters is wrong, it might still be possible to understand the meaning of the sentence even with the incorrect word. So too, a protein with a single incorrect amino acid might be able to work normally. It is also possible that with the mistyping, the meaning of the sentence will be quite different or even uninterpretable. The protein might work abnormally or not at all. Regardless of the outcome, this type of mutation is known as a missense mutation.

For example, the original sentence is "The quick brown fox jumps over the lazy dog." The new sentence might read "The qwick brown fox jumps over the lazy dog." The meaning is quite clear, even though there is a misspelling. "The quick brown fox **b**umps over the lazy dog." The sentence still makes sense, but the meaning is different. "The quick brown fox **m**umps over the lazy dog." The sentence no longer makes sense, grammatically or otherwise.

The third type of mutation is yet again confined to one position in the gene sequence and changes a single codon. But now the new codon is a stop codon. The ribosome will cut off the protein midway through the process of producing it. Just as a sentence with some of its words cut off isn't likely to make sense, it's likely that an incomplete, partial protein won't function at all. If it does function, it will function abnormally. This type of mutation is known as a nonsense mutation.

Using our example sentence, "The quick brown fox ju." There is not enough information here to make sense of it.

The fourth type of mutation results in either the deletion of base pairs from the DNA sequence or the insertion of base pairs. It is important to know whether the length of the insertion or deletion is a multiple of three. If so, the mutation will subtract or add full codons, which means subtracting amino acids from the protein or adding amino acids to it. Deleting letters or inserting random letters into the middle of a sentence is likely to change its meaning, but not always. Just so, a protein might still function normally if amino acids are subtracted or added.

Using our example sentence, "The quick fox jumps over the lazy dog," the meaning is mostly the same, despite the loss of the five letters in the word "brown." "The quick brown ox jumps over the lazy dog." The meaning is changed with the loss of one letter, but it is still understandable. "The quick brown over the lazy dog." The meaning is gone, with the loss of the three letters in the word "fox." "The quick fox jumps **c**over the lazy dog." With the addition of just one letter, the sentence no longer makes grammatical sense.

What happens if the length of the insertion or deletion in the DNA base pair sequence is not a multiple of three? Then all of the subsequent codons will be out of register, which will scramble all of the amino acids from that point onward. Imagine taking a sentence, picking a letter in the middle, and changing all of the subsequent letters to random letters. The effect on the sentence will very likely be profound. Similarly, the protein will not work properly, if at all. This is known as a frameshift mutation.

Using our example sentence: "The quick brown fop elyoa brp."

Armed with the knowledge of the different types of mutations that can occur in gene sequences and their potential consequences, let's consider the *KRIT1* mutation I'd found in my patient.

Murali had told me that there was a group of Hispanic families in the Southwestern United States with familial CCM. In my reading, I learned that a team of researchers had intensively studied the affected patients in those families. The researchers had speculated that these patients had a common ancestor, long ago. That ancestor had spontaneously developed the mutation in the *KRIT1* gene and then passed it down through the generations. If this thinking was correct, then many of the patients should have the same mutation in *KRIT1*, rather than them all having different mutations in the gene.

This is exactly what turned out to be the case. For most of the patients, the researchers found that in position 1363 of the *KRIT1* gene sequence, the normal cytosine base was altered to thymine in one of the two *KRIT1* copies in the genome (the other copy remained normal). This resulted in the normal CAA codon, which codes for the amino acid glutamine, becoming a TAA codon (transcribed to UAA in the messenger RNA), which is a stop codon. In other words, this is a nonsense mutation that results in only the first half of the protein being made. It was an open-and-shut case—

there was no question that this mutation affected the protein's function and was the cause of all of these patients' disease.

The mutation I had identified in my CCM patient was not so clear-cut. I'd found that in position 409 of the *KRIT1* gene sequence, the normal guanine base was altered to cytosine in one of the two *KRIT1* copies. The overlapping G and C peaks were clearly visible on the chromatogram (Figure 3). This mutation resulted in the normal GAT codon, which codes for the amino acid aspartate, becoming a CAT codon, which codes for the amino acid histidine. This was a missense mutation affecting the 137th amino acid in the protein. Was the aspartate changing to a histidine enough to interfere with the protein's normal function? I had no easy way to answer this question.

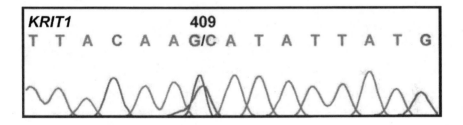

FIGURE 3

A return to the library and intensive reading of the scientific literature about *KRIT1* paid off. In the few years since the discovery of *KRIT1* as a gene responsible for familial CCM, a number of reports of specific *KRIT1* mutations identified in CCM patients had been published. I scoured through all of the reports I could find. No luck—none of them reported the same exact mutation I had discovered. But I did find a report of a different mutation that just happened to affect the same exact amino acid, the aspartate in the 137th position in the protein, and changed it into the amino acid glycine. It seemed too much to be a coincidence that two distinct missense mutations altering the same amino acid of the same protein would be identified in patients with the same disease. Perhaps it wasn't an open-and-shut case, but it was reasonably convincing. I concluded that I had identified the likely cause of the thousand holes in my patient's brain.

Unanswered in all of this was how the protein made from the *KRIT1* gene caused the disease. Not much was known about the protein's normal function, and why abnormal function would result in cavernomas appearing in the brain and spinal cord, and only in those locations. But that's how it goes. It is quite possible to achieve certainty that a mutated gene is responsible for a disease, without having any idea how that gene causes the disease. It can take researchers many more years or even decades to fully figure it out.

I was able to let the patient know that we thought we had identified the culprit gene and mutation responsible for his disease. He was pleased to find out about it, but the truth is that it didn't really change much of anything for him. We had already successfully addressed the patient's spinal mass with surgery, and his symptoms had improved. He and his wife were childless, and so there was no chance of his passing the *KRIT1* mutation on to future generations. We would never know if his sister had the mutation too. It is possible there were far-flung relatives who might have the mutation, but there was no way I was going to be able to track them down. The situation might have been different if the patient did have children; then we would want to test their DNA to see if any of them carried the *KRIT1* mutation. If any of them did, we might advise them to have a full neurological evaluation and have MRI scans of the brain and spinal cord to see if there were any problems brewing. But it wasn't as if we had a cure for the disease or a medical treatment to prevent cavernomas from forming and growing.

Despite these limitations, I came away feeling that my efforts on behalf of this one patient were fruitful. I had engaged with a person with a mysterious disease and come away with an explanation, touching his life in a small way. And, frankly, it had been a lot of fun to play medical detective. I caught a glimmer of what genetic medicine might look like in the future.

Since meeting the man with a thousand holes in his brain, I have done lots of DNA sequencing and looked at many thousands of chromatograms. Without a doubt the most striking chromatograms I have looked at in my career were in a manuscript I read fifteen years later, when I played detective again and used the chromatograms to judge whether humanity's first gene-edited babies—the first members of the CRISPR generation— had been born.

3

RISE OF THE GENETIC SUPERHEROES

When I was growing up during the 1980s, infection with the human immunodeficiency virus, widely known as HIV, was an automatic death sentence. Upon infection, the clock started ticking inexorably; the average time for progression to full-blown AIDS and death was about ten years. Even though there were quite a few other diseases killing far more people, the mysterious nature of HIV made it loom very large in the public's attention. I remember hearing far more about HIV and AIDS from my middle school science and health teachers (often conveyed in quasi-apocalyptic terms) than about heart disease and cancer.

By the 1990s, the development of HIV protease inhibitors was starting to turn HIV infection into a chronic condition rather than an invariably fatal one. But there was still an overwhelming need to find new ways to combat the virus. A small group of people who had been exposed to the HIV virus multiple times, in high-risk situations, yet had managed to evade infection were of intense interest to researchers. It seemed like these people had some sort of natural resistance or immunity to the virus. Might they have within their bodies the key to protecting the general population from HIV?

I first heard about the nature of that key during my first semester in the MD–PhD training program at Cornell University Medical Center and The Rockefeller University in 1997. My MD–PhD class had a weekly seminar series with lectures from prominent local physician-scientists. The idea was to provide us with role models who were equally comfortable treating patients at their bedsides and doing research at laboratory benches—and crossing between the two, bedside to bench and back, on a daily basis. One of our lecturers was Dr. Nathaniel Landau of the Aaron Diamond AIDS Research Center, known by the snappy acronym ADARC and affiliated with Rockefeller. Just in the past year, he had published a landmark paper in the HIV field. I hadn't been aware of the paper; at the time, my interest was in cancer and I tended to skip over the papers on infectious diseases when browsing through scientific journals. But as Dr. Landau explained the details of how his team had unraveled one cause of natural resistance to HIV, I listened with rapt attention.

HIV causes disease by hijacking and killing T cells, the sentinels of the immune system that circulate in the bloodstream and guard against infectious agents, both new foes and those the body has seen and fought off before. In particular, HIV targets a group of T cells that have a surface protein called CD4. The virus latches onto the CD4 protein and exploits it to gain entry into a cell, which it uses as a breeding ground for new viruses that kill the cell and go on to infect other cells. As HIV depletes these CD4-bearing cells, the human body loses its ability to fight off certain types of infections. These infections are the ultimate cause of death in AIDS, not the virus itself.

Landau and his colleagues at ADARC had been studying T cells from twenty-five HIV-resistant people. The T cells from two such individuals, code-named EU2 and EU3, particularly stood out. When isolated from their blood and exposed to HIV outside the body, these T cells needed to be treated with a thousand times more virus to become infected compared to T cells from regular people. Even after infection, the virus wasn't able to grow in the T cells. Clearly there was some special property inherent to the EU2 and EU3 T cells that made them resistant to HIV.

Earlier in 1996, six teams of researchers had reported that HIV needed more than just CD4 to infect T cells; at least one additional factor was involved. Each of the six teams had found that a protein called CCR5 could serve as that factor. Like CD4, CCR5 is a surface protein on T cells. When HIV attempts to enter a T cell, the virus extends a molecular finger called gp41 as a key to unlock a gate formed by the CD4 and CCR5 proteins together. Landau reasoned that there might be a problem with the CCR5 protein in the EU2 and EU3 T cells. He first looked at the overall amount of CCR5 protein in the resistant T cells compared to normal T cells. No difference. He then probed the gene that codes for the protein. When he used PCR to amplify the *CCR5* gene sequence out of the genome in either EU2 cells or EU3 cells, he found it to be significantly shorter than the normal version of the *CCR5* gene. Sanger sequencing determined that both the EU2 and EU3 versions of the gene had the exact same thirty-two-base pair deletion—a frameshift mutation—in the middle of the gene. Indeed, both EU2 and EU3 had the deletion in both copies of the *CCR5* gene in their genomes.

Because this deletion is thirty-two base pairs in length, a number that isn't a multiple of three, it won't cleanly remove amino acids from the CCR5 protein. Rather, it results in a scrambled string of amino acids starting at the location of the first affected codon. That portion of the normal protein, with each amino acid represented by a single letter abbreviation, looked like this:

...SSHFPYSQYQFWKNFQTLKIVILGLVLPLLVMVICYSGILK-TLLRCRNEKKRHRAV...

Whereas with the thirty-two-base pair deletion, looked like this (underline indicate differences):

...SSHFPY<u>IKDSHLGAGPAAACHGHLLLGNPKNSASVSK</u>.

It's not just that the amino acids are entirely mismatched. The period at the end of the second sequence denotes a stop codon, indicating that the protein ends much earlier than it should. A large portion of the protein is missing.

Landau investigated the effects of the deletion on the CCR5 protein and found that the defective protein was entirely missing from the cell surface. This meant the gate of entry used by HIV was no longer intact. No wonder, then, that the virus couldn't really infect the T cells. Landau then made a couple of additional important observations. When he sequenced the *CCR5* gene in a large number of people of European ancestry, he found that quite a few of them had the exact same thirty-two-base pair deletion on one of their two copies of the gene. (We now know that about ten percent of people of European ancestry have this mutation in one gene copy, and that about one percent have this mutation in both gene copies. But the mutation is largely absent from non-European populations.) And when he studied T cells from people with the deletion on only one gene copy, he found they could be infected quite readily with HIV, although the virus' growth was somewhat impaired. Having some but not all of the usual amount of normal CCR5 protein provided enough gates on the cell surface that HIV could still get into the cell.

Landau's remarkable study was published in August 2006 in the scientific journal *Cell*. Within weeks, two other teams of researchers reported this thirty-two-base pair deletion in *CCR5*, one in the journal *Science* and one in the journal *Nature*, though neither of the studies was as comprehensive as Landau's. Due to its prevalence in the population—at least in Europeans—the mutation became commonly known as *CCR5* delta32 or Δ32. It became clear that having two copies of *CCR5* Δ32 conferred high resistance to most strains of HIV (some strains are able to infect T cells by using proteins other than CCR5 as entry gates). Having one copy of the mutation didn't necessarily protect against an initial HIV infection, but it did seem to slow the progression of the disease from the initial infection to full-blown AIDS by a few years.

My classmates and I were wowed by Landau's lecture. In common parlance, the word mutation has a negative connotation, bringing to mind horrible diseases and sci-fi monsters. (It is for this reason that many researchers prefer to use a more neutral term like variant or polymorphism.) But some mutations can be beneficial to one's health. It seemed that EU2 and EU3, and other people with two copies of CCR5 Δ32, were like genetic superheroes—fortunate enough to have been born with an endowment of beneficial mutations from their parents.

Afterward, one of my classmates and I were chatting about Landau's work and wondering about its long-term implications. Wouldn't it be great, we thought, if you could put this mutation into an AIDS patient's T cells? It should cure their disease! This was immediately followed by the thought: we're only first-year medical students. If we can think of it, there's got to be lots of people who have already thought of it and are working on it.

Indeed, there were. Following the discovery of CCR5's role in HIV infection, at least seven companies attempted to develop a drug that blocks the interaction between the CCR5 protein and HIV's gp41. This would prevent HIV from opening the CD4/CCR5 gate and infecting the cell. The companies reasoned that since people lacking any working CCR5 protein—one percent of Europeans—are healthy, then a drug that blocks CCR5 should be safe. Only one such drug, maraviroc, has been fully developed so far. After proving to be effective in suppressing viral growth in patients in clinical trials, it was approved by the U.S. Food and Drug Administration in 2007.

Famously, one person has been cured of HIV through the direct effects of the CCR5 Δ32 mutation itself: the so-called Berlin patient. Timothy Ray Brown, an American, contracted the HIV virus in 1995. He was receiving standard antiviral medications when he was diagnosed with leukemia in 2006 while living in Berlin. After chemotherapy failed to treat the leukemia, his physician, Dr. Gero Hütter at the Charité Hospital in Berlin, recommended a bone marrow transplant. Hütter considered eighty potential bone marrow donors who were an immunological match with Brown. Reasoning that it might be possible to treat both Brown's leukemia and HIV infection simultaneously (the bone marrow is the source of all of a person's T cells), Hütter screened the potential donors for the *CCR5 Δ 32* mutation and identified a donor who had two copies of the mutation. Brown underwent a transplant with that donor's bone marrow and stopped taking antiviral therapy.

By sixty days after the transplant, all of Brown's T cells showed the double Δ32 mutation, and the HIV virus couldn't be detected in his blood. Unfortunately, Brown suffered a recurrence of the leukemia less than a year after the transplant. Hütter arranged for a second bone marrow transplant from the same donor. The repeat transplant worked, and a decade later Brown remained in remission from the leukemia and showed no signs of active HIV virus in his body, despite never again taking antiviral medications after the first transplant. Brown was considered by physicians to have achieved a complete cure, the first one ever.

This success story validates the strategy of using lessons learned from people who have won the genetic lottery—by inheriting beneficial mutations from their parents—to help those who aren't so lucky. Unfortunately, Brown's cure has not proven as successful in other patients. Bone marrow transplants are very risky, and most patients receiving double-Δ32 bone marrow transplants to cure both leukemia and HIV have died from complications of the procedure. Those surviving their transplants have had their HIV infections surge again, apparently due to the virus adapting so it doesn't need the CCR5 protein to infect T cells. Nonetheless, the story of the Berlin patient has inspired other approaches to introduce beneficial *CCR5* mutations into HIV patients. And the implications of the story certainly have not been lost on researchers and physicians who are trying to combat other common diseases, like heart disease.

The first time I learned about the *PCSK9* gene was before it even had a name. At the annual retreat of my MD–PhD training program in the summer of 2002, my classmate Kara Maxwell was giving a talk about her work in the Rockefeller laboratory of Dr. Jan Breslow, a world authority on cholesterol. Maxwell had been doing experiments in which she fed some mice with high-cholesterol diets and other mice with low-cholesterol diets. She was using a relatively new technology, gene chips, that could measure the relative amounts of messenger RNAs transcribed from all the genes in the genome. She had applied the gene chips to liver samples from her mice and analyzed the data to see which genes were most affected by the addition of cholesterol to the diet.

Maxwell had found that after just one day of exposure to high cholesterol, several genes had reduced transcription. Most of these genes coded for proteins involved in cholesterol production. This made perfect sense. When the liver detects that there's not enough cholesterol coming into the body through the diet, it has the ability to pick up the slack by making cholesterol molecules from scratch. Conversely, if there is enough (or too much) cholesterol in the body, the liver dials down its production. Maxwell noticed there was another gene that was reduced, a gene that had never been studied before. It was so obscure that it was only known by a meaningless database number: AI747682. Maxwell speculated that this gene might code for a previously unknown protein involved in cholesterol production. Whatever it was, it seemed likely to be important.

Dr. Nabil Seidah at the Clinical Research Institute of Montreal in Canada came upon this same gene by a totally different path. He had been studying a family of proteins called proprotein convertases, which were enzymes that cleaved other proteins and turned them from inactive forms into active forms. He was trawling through the human, mouse, and rat genomes looking for new members of this family. He was able to track one down, the ninth protein of its kind; although it was originally known as NARC-1, he would soon come to call it proprotein convertase subtilisin/kexin type 9, or PCSK9. Seidah published his work on this gene in February 2003. On seeing his paper, Maxwell realized it was the same gene she had been studying.

Not long afterward, yet another group of researchers converged upon this gene, this time through genetics. Drs. Marianne Abifadel and Catherine Boileau at Necker-Enfants Malades Hospital in Paris had been studying French patients with sky-high levels of LDL cholesterol—the bad kind of cholesterol that puts people at risk for heart disease, specifically coronary artery disease, which causes heart attacks. These patients had levels so high they were suffering heart attacks as early as childhood. The condition seemed to run in families, so they were diagnosed with the disease known as familial hypercholesterolemia. None of the known cholesterol genes seemed to be involved. So Abifadel and Boileau were on the hunt for something new. Through painstaking work, they mapped the responsible gene to one particular region of chromosome 1. With Sanger sequencing of various genes in that region, they realized the patients had mutations in the recently named *PCSK9* gene. After conferring with Seidah, they published their discovery in a brief paper in June 2003. One question they weren't able to answer: did the patient mutations hobble the coded protein, or did the mutations actually make the protein work better than normal, which is to say, hyperactively?

Maxwell and Seidah were both well positioned to answer that question, as each had already been studying the gene. They independently used a virus to carry the gene into the livers of mice, which had the effect of pumping up the production of the PCSK9 protein. They both observed that the mice's LDL cholesterol levels shot up in response to the increased protein. This established that the patient mutations causing familial hypercholesterolemia were making the protein hyperactive. Subsequent work showed that the PCSK9 protein was mostly produced in the liver and then exported into the bloodstream, where it seemed to be blocking the removal of LDL cholesterol from the bloodstream. It was a simple relationship: more PCSK9 equals more LDL cholesterol equals a higher risk of heart disease. I got to hear it all from Maxwell firsthand before I graduated from our MD–PhD program in the summer of 2004.

I didn't think about PCSK9 again for another couple of years, and it happened in a most unusual way. I had moved to Boston to do my medical internship and residency at Brigham and Women's Hospital. One morning in the summer of 2005, I was on rounds in the medical intensive care unit after. doing an overnight shift taking care of the very sick patients in the unit. The rounds were an opportunity for the outgoing night medical team to discuss each patient in detail with the incoming day medical team and make sure that everyone was on the same page as to the next steps in the patients' care. Normally the teams' attention was squarely focused on the person presenting the patients, which on this occasion happened to be me.

Right as I was about to start on one of the patient presentations, I received a message on my pager: "Please call – Marshall."

Uh oh. Normally I would put off answering pages until after rounds were over. I couldn't leave a dozen of my colleagues standing around, waiting on me, while we were in the middle of rounds. But when I showed everyone the page, they immediately understood that this couldn't wait.

Dr. Marshall Wolf had been the director of the internal medicine residency program at Brigham and Women's Hospital for decades and, even after he stepped down to take a more senior leadership position at the hospital, was still the heart and soul of the program. He was also an inscrutable man, even at the best of times. When I had interviewed for my internship at the Brigham, one of my meetings was with Wolf. It was easily the most awkward interview I have had in my career. I had no idea what was going on in his head, but I had the unsettling feeling that he could see right through me, with all of my faults laid bare. He referred to things about my life that he really shouldn't have had any way of knowing. I left his office absolutely certain that I had bombed the interview. But he must have liked me. Otherwise there's no way I would have ended up at the Brigham for my internship and residency. Still, to get a terse page from Wolf now, out of the blue—it was either good news, or I was in big trouble.

I broke away from rounds, went to the closest phone, and gave him a call.

Wolf immediately answered and, skipping the pleasantries, went straight to the point. "I just met with John Maraganore, the CEO of Alnylam," he said. "His company works on RNA. I remember that you worked on RNA for your PhD. I think it's a great opportunity for you. He's expecting your call."

Even if I hadn't been running on fumes after an overnight shift in the unit, this would have been hard for me to unpack. When I timidly asked for clarification, he said, "you should consult for them. Just get in touch with John. Here's his number." End conversation.

Had Wolf really just set up a consulting arrangement for me with a biotechnology company? I couldn't wrap my head around it. But I went on with rounds, and after having a chance to recover from the night's work, I got in touch with Maraganore, half expecting he would have no idea who I was. But he knew exactly who I was. "Marshall said wonderful things about you," he told me. "I'd love to meet with you over coffee in the next few weeks."

When I met with Maraganore, he told me that Alnylam was trying to develop therapeutics using the new technology of RNA interference. Originally discovered by Dr. Andrew Fire at the Carnegie Institution of Science and Dr. Craig Mello at the University of Massachusetts Medical School (an accomplishment for which they'd receive the Nobel Prize in Physiology or Medicine in 2006), RNA interference took advantage of a natural phenomenon in which a short double-strand RNA molecule with a sequence matching a portion of a messenger RNA would cause that messenger RNA to be destroyed by the cell. Alnylam's plan was to synthesize these short RNA molecules, deliver them into the body, and silence disease-causing genes. They now had the technology working pretty well, especially in the liver, so it was time to start thinking about which diseases to go after. Mara-ganore thought that someone like myself, still in training and on the front line of medicine, would be in the best position to advise on unmet medical needs that could be addressed by RNA interference.

It sounded good, and I entered into a consulting arrangement with Alnylam, even though I was skeptical that I would be of much help. But Maraganore's instincts turned out to be right on. Later that year, I took care of a hospitalized patient, in his 50s, with heart failure from a condition called cardiac amyloidosis. It is caused by a protein called transthyretin that is produced only by the liver (from a gene called *TTR*) and exported into the bloodstream. In some patients, the transthyretin forms clumps (called amyloid) while in the blood and then ends up getting trapped in organs like the heart and nerves. As the clumps build up in the organs, they can cause life-threatening problems.

My patient was in exactly that situation. His heart was so thickened with amyloid clumps that his only recourse was getting a heart transplant. I was shepherding him through the process of being evaluated as a trans-plant candidate. It required a whole battery of tests to make sure that if he did receive a heart he would live long enough for it to be worthwhile. Donor hearts being a very scarce resource, it was absolutely critical to make sure they went to the patients who could most benefit from them.

The patient was a super friendly, engaging man, and I found that I liked him immensely. So it was heartbreaking when one of the scans showed a probable tumor in his liver. Any concern for cancer meant he was disqualified from getting a heart transplant. Unfortunately, there were no other treatments for cardiac amyloidosis. We would just have to manage his heart failure as best we could, with the understanding that he didn't have much time left to live.

As I learned and thought more about cardiac amyloidosis, I real-ized that it might represent the perfect application of Alnylam's technology. There was a great unmet need—besides a heart transplant, there was no existing treatment. The offending protein was produced in the liver, where Alnylam could deliver their technology. Transthyretin didn't seem to have any essential purpose in the body, so if the *TTR* gene was silenced by RNA interference, there shouldn't be any serious side effects. If transthyretin production was cut off at the source, it'd mean no transthyretin in the blood, which would mean no amyloid clumps. It's possible that given time, the clumps already in the heart might get cleared out. Even if that didn't happen, the treatment might still stop the condition from getting worse.

I made my recommendation to the team at Alnylam, where it seemed to be well received. I didn't find out about it until a few years later, but after further considering amyloidosis and consulting with specialists for the disease, Alnylam decided to make it the company's lead drug development program. Fast forward a little more than a decade later, August 2018. After clinical trials proved its ability to reduce transthyretin production and to improve patients' quality of life, patisiran was approved by the U.S. Food and Drug Administration. It was the very first RNA-interference drug.

Having offered up amyloidosis as a possible therapeutic opportunity in the spring of 2006, I was thinking about other diseases that involve the liver. It was right around this time that Drs. Jonathan Cohen and Helen Hobbs at the University of Texas Southwestern Medical Center published a landmark study on *PCSK9* in the *New England Journal of Medicine*, a true game-changer.

Cohen and Hobbs had been intrigued by the finding that increased *PCSK9* activity caused familial hypercholesterolemia. Mutations that cause a protein to be hyperactive are quite unusual; mutations that inactivate a protein are much more common. It's much easier to break something than it is to make it work better than normal. So there were probably some inactivating *PCSK9* mutations out there in the population waiting to be found, they reasoned. Since the hyperactive mutations increased LDL cholesterol, presumably the inactivating mutations would decrease LDL cholesterol. They sequenced the *PCSK9* gene in 128 people with low LDL cholesterol—

half African Americans, half European Americans—and hit pay dirt. They identified two different *PCSK9* nonsense mutations among the African Americans, each mutation resulting in a defective protein.

When Cohen and Hobbs looked for these same nonsense mutations in a larger group of several thousand African Americans, they found that three percent of them carried one copy of one of the mutations. Remarkably, these lucky three percent not only had about a thirty percent reduction in LDL cholesterol levels, they also had about a ninety percent reduction in the risk of coronary artery disease! Their *PCSK9* nonsense mutations had turned them into genetic superheroes.

The story became even more exciting when Cohen and Hobbs reported a few months later that they'd identified a woman with inactivating mutations in both copies of *PCSK9*, who had no working PCSK9 protein at all. She was in her thirties, in excellent health, an aerobics instructor, with two children—despite her LDL cholesterol being jaw-droppingly low. South African researchers later identified a healthy woman with no working PCSK9 protein and with a rock-bottom LDL cholesterol level in Zimbabwe. These two women made it abundantly clear that *PCSK9* wasn't required for good health.

Because the PCSK9 protein is largely produced in the liver and then exported into the bloodstream, it was an opportunity tailor-made for Alnylam's technology. Just as with transthyretin, PCSK9 protein in the bloodstream could be greatly reduced by silencing its genetic source in the liver with RNA interference. That should result in lower LDL cholesterol and lower risk of heart disease, just as was seen with the naturally occurring *PCSK9* nonsense mutations. And the existence of healthy people who lacked PCSK9 altogether suggested that a drug targeting *PCSK9* would be safe. It was a no-brainer.

I was involved in several meetings at Alnylam in which we debated which groups of patients would benefit from a *PCSK9* drug, but there was no question that the gene was worth pursuing. Alnylam soon launched a

development program around *PCSK9*. After a decade of work, the resulting drug, inclisiran, has proven highly effective and safe at reducing LDL
cholesterol levels in heart disease patients in clinical trials. The drug appears
to be on track for approval by the U.S. Food and Drug Administration.

Alnylam wasn't the only company that took an interest in *PCSK9*.
Many other pharmaceutical companies have at least dipped their toes
into the water. Several companies decided to go after the PCSK9 protein
directly in the bloodstream. They created synthetic antibodies that grab
PCSK9 and neutralize it, modeled on naturally occurring human antibodies that fight off infections. Two such antibodies, alirocumab and evolo-
cumab, received approval from the U.S. Food and Drug Administration
in 2015. Over the next few years, large clinical trials showed both drugs to
reduce the risk of heart problems in high-risk patients.

But these drugs haven't proven to be as popular as originally
expected. For starters, the companies decided to charge exorbitant prices
for the drugs—more than $14,000 per year—which led to reluctance
among insurers to pay for prescriptions. The dosing regimen is also an
impediment for patients. Each drug needs to be injected under the skin,
every few weeks, for the rest of the patient's life. An unattractive proposition compared to swallowing a pill every day, which is the case with statin
drugs, the traditional way to lower cholesterol. Despite these issues, *PCSK9*
is widely regarded as a success story for genetics: just twelve years between
the gene's discovery and the approval of medications for use in patients.

Yet another group of genetic superheroes came to light because of a
deliberate search for them. In late 2009, the new technique called exome
sequencing was very much on my mind. Dr. Jay Shendure at the University
of Washington in Seattle had recently published a landmark paper reporting the very first use of exome sequencing on DNA samples from human
beings. Shendure had been a student in Harvard Medical School's combined

MD–PhD training program. Our paths had crossed while he was finishing medical school; he was assigned to my internal medicine team for a few weeks while I was a resident at Brigham and Women's Hospital. We chatted at length about the pros and cons of doing additional medical training— internship, residency, even a fellowship—versus committing to full-time research. He chose the latter. After graduating, he took a faculty position at the University of Washington in 2007 and went straight to work.

Exome sequencing entails determining the base pair sequences of all of the protein-coding portions of DNA in the thousands of genes in the human genome—about two percent of the genome, when they're added up. It takes advantage of so-called next-generation sequencing. Instead of laboriously doing Sanger sequencing for each small stretch of DNA, a few hundred base pairs at a time, next-generation sequencing allows one to simply collect all of the DNA one wishes to sequence in one batch and feed it into a machine. The machine can do massively parallel sequencing of millions or even billions of base pairs all at one time. This dramatically reduces the time and expense of doing large-scale sequencing. The Human Genome Project, which relied on Sanger sequencing, required thirteen years and $3 billion to sequence the first genome in its entirety. Next-generation sequencing can now do a full human genome in less than twenty-four hours for a few hundred U.S. dollars.

In 2009, next-generation sequencing was still expensive. Most disease-causing mutations of interest to researchers, physicians, and patients directly affect proteins—missense, nonsense, and frameshift mutations—so it made sense to sequence only the two percent of the genome in the exome, rather than the full genome. Shendure's innovation was to capture and purify that two percent out of a sample of full genomic DNA. He could then focus the next-generation sequencing on just that two percent. In his initial report published in *Nature* in September 2009, he applied exome sequencing to DNA samples from twelve people, including four patients with a disease called Freeman–Sheldon syndrome. With the exome sequencing data from the four patients, he was able to tie

Freeman–Sheldon syndrome to mutations in the *MYH3* gene. This gene's association with the syndrome was already known. But a few months later, Shendure used his exome sequencing platform to discover the previously unknown cause of another disease called Miller syndrome: mutations in the *DHODH* gene.

At the time, I was doing a postdoctoral research fellowship at the Broad Institute in Cambridge, Massachusetts, having recently finished my training as a clinical cardiologist with a focus on the prevention of coronary artery disease. The Broad Institute was ramping up to do exome sequencing at a large scale. The sequencing team was in the process of completing exomes from sixty cancer patients and had the capacity to do more. They were amenable to doing exome sequencing for an additional handful of patient DNA samples, if offered a compelling reason.

Dr. Sekar Kathiresan, one of my postdoctoral research advisors, and I were having one of our regular chats when the conversation turned to exome sequencing. We brainstormed about how to get the most bang for the buck out of exome sequencing, given the cost. We thought that a family with an inherited disease, of unknown cause, might be a good place to start. We could do exome sequencing for a few of the affected family members and see if there was a gene mutation shared by all of them. That mutation could be the cause of the disease. But then, we thought, why did it have to be a disease? Maybe it could be an inherited condition that was actually beneficial. People who'd inherited rock-bottom LDL cholesterol levels would be protected from heart disease, we reasoned. So perhaps we should look for families with such people.

We realized the easiest way to look was by simply reading the scientific literature. We came across a series of papers written by Dr. Gustav Schonfeld at Washington University in St. Louis. Schonfeld had been a survivor of the Nazi concentration camp at Auschwitz during his childhood and settled in St. Louis after World War II. He'd gone on to have a distinguished career as a physician-scientist who specialized in cholesterol disorders. He'd described a family with members who had a condition called familial hypobetalipoproteinemia, which is medical jargon meaning a very low LDL cholesterol level. One of the family members had come to his attention after she had attended a health fair organized by her employer and had her cholesterol levels checked. Her LDL cholesterol was so astonishingly low that she was referred to Schonfeld's clinic for further evaluation, even though she was in excellent health. He recruited her as well as many of her family members into a research study to attempt to discover the gene responsible for her condition.

Despite his best efforts over the course of a decade, Schonfeld had been unable to pinpoint the gene. He was limited by the research techniques available at the time. The best he was able to do was figure out that the gene was on chromosome 1. As of 2009, it remained an unsolved case.

After reviewing Schonfeld's papers closely, Kathiresan and I were excited that we'd found a perfect scenario for exome sequencing. We could use brute force to figure out the right gene—sequence all twenty-thousand protein-coding genes and see which one had mutations that explained the low LDL cholesterol. The family was large, spread across three generations, and it looked like Schonfeld had studied DNA samples from thirty-eight family members. The only question was whether Schonfeld would be willing to share the samples. So Kathiresan reached out to him. It turned out that Schonfeld had recently retired, but the DNA samples were safely stored away in a freezer on the university campus. It'd be no problem to have someone track them down and ship them to us.

Schonfeld was also kind enough to share all of the data he had on the family members. I spent a full day carefully going over the data and realized something even more interesting than advertised was going on. It wasn't just LDL cholesterol that was involved. Quite a few of the family members had low LDL cholesterol and many of them also had low triglycerides (the fat content in cholesterol-carrying particles in the bloodstream). But four siblings in the second generation (one of whom was the woman identified at the health fair) also had very low HDL cholesterol, the good form of cholesterol. Nobody else in the family had abnormal HDL cholesterol. Furthermore, the four siblings had the lowest LDL cholesterol and triglyceride levels in the entire family.

Those four siblings were the key to the puzzle. Their parents didn't seem to be as severely affected. When seen in a family, this is a clue that the condition is caused by two mutations, one in each of the two copies of the gene (one from the mother and one from the father). We realized that by exome sequencing the DNA samples from just two of the four siblings, we might be able to crack the case. We just needed to find one gene, out of the twenty-thousand genes in the genome, that had two mutations in both of the siblings.

This was fortunate, because the Broad Institute's sequencing team was able to process only two of our DNA samples. We picked the two siblings who had the lowest combination of LDL cholesterol, HDL cholesterol, and triglycerides. Because all three measurements were low, and we couldn't find any previous description of this triple-combo in the scientific literature, we decided to give the condition a name that admittedly was pure jargon: familial combined hypolipidemia.

At this point I teamed up with two students who'd recently joined Kathiresan's team—James Pirruccello, a medical student visiting from Johns Hopkins University School of Medicine, and Ron Do, a graduate student visiting from McGill University in Canada. Our job was to figure out how to process and interpret the exome sequencing data once the Broad Institute generated it. Exome sequencing was so new that the Broad Institute didn't have a standard computational pipeline yet. We would have to jury-rig our own pipeline.

During the first couple of months of 2010, Pirruccello and Do did a masterful job of setting up various pieces of the pipeline and getting them all to play nicely with each other. By the time the Broad Institute's sequencing team had the exome sequencing data ready, the pipeline was ready to go. On Friday, February 19, Pirruccello set the pipeline running. By late Saturday morning, the pipeline had finished its run. Pirruccello emailed me to let me know that something interesting had showed up. We agreed to meet in person shortly afterward. It didn't matter in the slightest that it was a weekend afternoon. (Though it turned out that Do, being perhaps more athletically minded than Pirruccello and me, was at the gym.) We had been working toward this goal for a few months, and now it was time to see if it had paid off.

It had.

Pirruccello and I started going over the data spit out by the pipeline. Pirruccello directed my attention to one of the most interesting findings: a gene called *ANGPTL3*. It'd been flagged as having a nonsense mutation in one copy of the gene. A GAA codon (coding for the amino acid glutamine) was changed to a TAA codon (stop codon). Although there was no reason to think that the mutations we were looking for would be nonsense mutations—they just as easily could have been missense mutations—we were keenly aware that a nonsense mutation or a frameshift mutation was almost certain to kill a protein's activity. The effect of a missense mutation was much harder to predict. So of course we looked for any nonsense or frameshift mutations first. There was something funny about *ANGPTL3*, though. It turned out to have not one, not two, but three mutations. One more than we were looking for.

We didn't know what to make of this. Neither the second mutation nor the third mutation was a nonsense or frameshift mutation. The second was TCC (serine) to TGC (cysteine). Potentially interesting, since it was a missense mutation. The third was TCC (serine) to TCA (serine). Not at all interesting, since it didn't actually change the amino acid. Then we noticed that the second and third mutations were in the same part of the gene, right next to each other.

It took us only a moment to come to an electrifying realization. They weren't two separate mutations—it was a single mutation that affected two adjacent DNA base pairs, which was unusual, but not unheard of. And when we put the two changes together: TCC (serine) to TGA (stop codon). It was a second nonsense mutation in *ANGPTL3*!

This was a scientific smoking gun if ever there was one. The two siblings shared two different nonsense mutations in *ANGPTL3*, one inherited from each parent. They'd have no functional ANGPTL3 protein because of their naturally occurring mutations. They'd be what geneticists call knockouts. There was no question in our minds—this had to be the right gene.

The dominoes then fell in rapid succession. We realized that *ANGPTL3* was located on chromosome 1, exactly where Schonfeld had predicted it would be. When we did a quick search of the scientific literature, we saw that the gene had been discovered eleven years earlier as being the cause of low triglycerides in mice. The coded protein was produced exclusively in the liver and secreted into the bloodstream, where it turned off an enzyme that metabolized triglycerides. Nobody had connected the gene to LDL cholesterol, though, for the simple reason that mice don't make much LDL cholesterol to begin with.

Only fifteen minutes had passed, but one hundred percent convinced we had the answer, we knew we needed to share the news with Kathiresan without delay. (Do was still at the gym, and we didn't connect with him until later in the day.) Kathiresan was every bit as excited as we were. By the end of the afternoon, after multiple phone conversations, we'd hatched our plan. We'd confirm the two nonsense mutations using Sanger sequencing. We would test all thirty-eight family members to see who had none, one, or both of the mutations. And we would start working on a manuscript without delay. We of course let Schonfeld know the good news as well. He was pleased to see the biggest cold case left over from his long, productive career finally solved. (Sadly, Schonfeld passed away the following year.)

Over the next week, we confirmed the mutations and tracked them in the family. It turned out that one of the mutations was already in the family, and then a man with the other mutation married into the family and had ten children, including the four siblings with familial combined hypolipidemia. These four were the only ones in the family who had both mutations. And as far as we could tell, they seemed to be in perfect health— no ill effects whatsoever from having no working *ANGPTL3* at all.

With these results in hand, we rushed to finish the study, working around the clock. On a Sunday afternoon soon afterward, I was working on the manuscript with Do and Pirruccello in an empty cafeteria in the research building. The Winter Olympics were underway in Vancouver, and we had the television on in the background, showing the gold medal game of the men's hockey tournament, Canada versus the United States. As a Canadian, Do was fervently rooting for his team to win; as Americans, Pirruccello and I were just as heartily supporting our team. Our work came to a halt as the game went to overtime. When the Canadian team ended up scoring the winning goal in thrilling fashion, I couldn't help but feel happy for Do. Even though my team had lost, our exuberance about the *ANGPTL3* story meant there were plenty of good feelings to go around.

From the day we learned about the *ANGPTL3* mutations to the day we submitted the manuscript to the *New England Journal of Medicine*, the premiere medical journal, was just nineteen days. The paper was published later that year. But it left a very important question unanswered: do *ANGPTL3* mutations protect against heart disease? It seemed like low LDL cholesterol and low triglycerides should be a good thing. But the burden of proof was on us. And it ended up taking Kathiresan and me seven years to prove our case.

To show a protective effect of *ANGPTL3* mutations, we needed to show that they occurred more frequently in healthy people than in patients with coronary artery disease. The problem was that unlike *PCSK9*, for which mutations occur in three percent of the population, *ANGPTL3* mutations are much rarer, about one in three hundred people. What ended up making it possible to do our analysis was exome sequencing studies and

DNA chip studies of tens of thousands of people, funded in large part by the U.S. National Institutes of Health. Because these studies assessed all of the twenty-thousand genes in the human genome, it was straightforward to extract data for just the gene of interest to us, *ANGPTL3*. We had to do some additional work to decipher whether the *ANGPTL3* missense mutations we found inactivated the protein or not. In the end, we were able to conclude that inactivating *ANGPTL3* mutations reduce the risk of coronary artery disease by more than a third. There's evidence too that the same mutations reduce the risk of type 2 diabetes.

Our work over the last decade has found that *ANGPTL3* mutations are what we think of as a quadruple-whammy: lower LDL cholesterol, lower triglycerides, lower risk of heart disease, and lower risk of diabetes. And there appears to be no downside to having a single *ANGPTL3* mutation, or even having two *ANGPTL3* mutations. Not surprisingly, pharmaceutical companies have taken notice. There are at least three companies actively developing *ANGPTL3* therapies, and so far their drugs have performed well in clinical trials, reducing both LDL cholesterol and triglycerides in volunteers and patients.

Three genes—*CCR5*, *PCSK9*, *ANGPTL3*—have emerged as compelling drug targets after being discovered to have inactivating mutations that protect against disease. More such genes are coming out of the woodwork. It's only natural to wonder whether it'd be possible to recreate these naturally occurring mutations in the rest of the population, those not fortunate enough to have won the genetic lottery. If you had the chance to become a genetic superhero, or to ensure your child was a genetic superhero, would you take that chance?

With gene editing, you might have that chance not too far in the future.

4

THE DECADES-LONG BIRTH OF GENE EDITING

Imagine that you have just discovered a new gene linked to a disease you're studying. You made this discovery by harnessing the tools of modern genetics, perhaps by doing exome sequencing in family members with the disease. You are now facing the problem that you don't know anything about the gene—how it operates in the human body, much less how mutations in the gene cause the disease. What would you do next?

Typically, you would take advantage of the fact that most genes are shared among many species. This is especially true for closely related species. For humans, this means the full spectrum of mammals. Researchers frequently use one particular mammal as a proxy for humans, as a model animal in which to study human diseases—the species *Mus musculus*, more commonly known as the house mouse. Mice are related closely enough to humans that the function of a gene in humans will be very similar to the function of the same gene in mice. Mice offer other advantages. They breed relatively quickly, with the full span of pregnancy being just three weeks. They have also been studied so extensively by so many researchers for decades that there are well-established methods to modify genes in mice.

The classic approach is to use a special kind of mouse cell called embryonic stem cells. As the name implies, these cells originate from mouse embryos. Embryos represent the very first stage of life before birth. When an egg cell from a mother and a sperm cell from a father unite in the process called fertilization, they form a single cell known as a zygote. This single cell has the potential to become a full-grown mouse. What this means is that after the single cell divides and divides and divides into a large number of cells, they diversify into a wide variety of cell types—hundreds in total, including muscle cells, liver cells, fat cells, red and white blood cells, and egg or sperm cells, to name just a few—that make up all of the different organs in the mouse's body. In scientific parlance, the zygote is pluripotent.

It turns out that the single-cell zygote is not the only cell that's pluripotent. After the zygote divides, it becomes two cells. One more round of division yields four cells. After another round, eight cells. A few more rounds take the count up to a few hundred cells. At that stage of the embryo's growth, some of the cells are still pluripotent. Each has the potential to give rise to any of the cell types in any of the organs in the body.

Why is this important? The pluripotent cells can be isolated from mouse embryos and coaxed into growing in a dish in the laboratory indefinitely. They keep dividing, and dividing, and dividing—becoming millions or even billions of cells—and they remain pluripotent. Drs. Martin Evans and Matthew Kaufman at the University of Cambridge and, independently, Dr. Gail Martin at the University of California, San Francisco, were the first to achieve this feat, reported in 1981. These researchers took advantage of a technique called in vitro fertilization, uniting a mouse egg cell and a mouse sperm cell into a zygote in the laboratory and then allowing the zygote to develop into an embryo in a dish. In the proper conditions, the embryo could be maintained outside a mother's body for more than a week. (It could also be frozen and stored indefinitely.) This made it easier to harvest the pluripotent cells from the embryos and grow them into so-called embryonic stem cells.

In vitro fertilization is the same technique that's used to make human embryos outside the body, usually for the purpose of assisted reproduction for infertile couples. After the embryos are made, they can be transferred into a mother's uterus to establish a pregnancy and then brought to term. The embryos' unusual origins are the reason the live-born offspring are known as test tube babies.

Over the next few years, Evans' team of researchers tested whether their mouse embryonic stem cells could be placed back into a new mouse embryo made by in vitro fertilization. They indeed could get the stem cells to fully incorporate into the embryo and, being pluripotent, contribute all of the different cell types to the adult's body. The resulting adult mouse was a chimera, named after the hybrid lion-goat-snake creature of Greek mythology. Because the embryo was a mix of the original cells and the added embryonic stem cells, some of the cells in the adult derived from the original cells, and the remainder of the cells derived from the embryonic stem cells. For the next step, Evans' team used viruses to slip foreign DNA into the genome in mouse embryonic stem cells, permanently marking those cells. The researchers then added the marked stem cells into new mouse embryos, which after pregnancy and birth became chimeric mice in which the foreign DNA was present in many different cell types in the body. Evans' team had found a roundabout way to insert DNA sequences into living animals. This accomplishment opened the door to modifying the mouse's own genes.

In parallel during the 1980s, Dr. Mario Capecchi at the University of Utah and Dr. Oliver Smithies at the University of Wisconsin–Madison were independently trying to modify genes in mouse embryonic stem cells. They each worked out a process called homologous recombination, in which a stretch of DNA sequence in the genome in a cell could be replaced with a synthetic version of the same DNA sequence in which some desired changes had been made. The synthetic version was made in the laboratory and slipped into cells. As long as there was enough matching between the native DNA sequence and the synthetic DNA sequence, a spontaneous swapping could occur, tricking the cell into taking the desired changes into its genome. That something like this could happen might have seemed like magic. But the process proved to be extremely inefficient—for every million cells where this was attempted, perhaps one cell would get the desired changes. Not good odds at all.

But there was a clever trick to improve the efficiency of homologous recombination: use an antibiotic drug that ordinarily was lethal to mouse embryonic stem cells. A foreign gene that created resistance to the antibiotic was placed in the synthetic DNA sequence. Any cell that swapped in the synthetic DNA sequence would now survive exposure to the antibiotic. It didn't work perfectly, but after the antibiotic killed off all of the unchanged cells, the proportion of correctly modified cells went from one in a million cells to perhaps one in one hundred cells. This was good enough that researchers could find the desired one cell out of the one hundred cells without too much work.

By the late 1980s, the work of Evans, Capecchi, and Smithies had converged to make it possible to generate so-called knockout mice, in which a gene had been inactivated and permanently turned off. The same approach made it possible to generate knock-in mice, in which a mutation was either inserted into a gene or, if the original gene already had a mutation, in which the mutation was corrected.

Researchers could now carry out an extended sequence of steps to make gene-modified mice. They could grow mouse embryonic stem cells in the laboratory; use homologous recombination to inactivate a gene, introduce a specific mutation into a gene, or correct a gene mutation in a cell's genome; grow the gene-modified stem cell into a large number of cells; add some of those cells into mouse embryos; use the embryos to establish pregnancies; and await the birth of mice in which some (but not all) cells had the gene modification. The resulting mice would be chimeras. It would be hoped that some of the egg cells or sperm cells in the chimeras were derived from the added stem cells and would therefore carry the gene modification. If so, breeding of the chimeras with other mice might yield some offspring that carried the gene modification in all of their cells—full knockout or knock-in mice.

In 1989, four different teams of researchers were the first to use the methods pioneered by Evans, Capecchi, and Smithies to generate gene-modified mice. Many more successful demonstrations soon followed. It's not a quick or easy process—it typically takes one to two years from start to finish. Even so, thousands of different gene-modified mice have been made with these methods. No surprise, then, that the trio of scientists received the Nobel Prize in Physiology or Medicine in 2007.

The ability to make gene-modified mice has revolutionized biomedical research. If a specific gene mutation has been linked to disease in humans, then it's often possible to make knock-in mice with the analogous mutation. If those mice have a disease similar to the human disease, then researchers can intensively study the disease in the mice in a way that's not possible in humans, due to ethical principles of human medical research. Researchers can test experimental therapies in the gene-modified mice as a way of getting important information about the effectiveness and safety of the therapies before planning any clinical trials involving human patients.

But there are times when mice aren't good enough. It might be that a human disease gene isn't present in mice. It might be that a human mutation has no correlation in the mouse genome. It might be that when it comes to the disease in question, human biology is simply too different from mouse biology. What to do then?

I found myself facing this very question as I was starting my postdoctoral fellowship at Massachusetts General Hospital and the Broad Institute, both in the Boston area, in the summer of 2008. Having just completed my training in clinical cardiology, I was keen to tackle coronary artery disease, the leading cause of death in the world. In the wake of the Human

Genome Project, it was now possible to scan the entire human genome to find new genetic factors involved in heart attacks. Some interesting candidates were emerging. But some of the candidates were nowhere to be found in the mouse genome. Worse, mice don't get coronary artery disease or suffer heart attacks. So making knockout or knock-in mice wasn't really an option.

This got me thinking hard about an alternative solution. First and foremost, I needed to study cells with a human genome. Where better to study genetic factors originally discovered in the human genome? Then I needed the ability to make genetic modifications in the cells. Finally, I needed to be able to study the cell types involved in various aspects of cardiovascular disease—the vascular cells in blood vessels, heart muscle cells, and liver cells, for starters. But experimental modification of the genome in cells in a living human being, even if it were possible, would be a non-starter for ethical reasons. The only alternative would be to work with cells in a dish in the laboratory. So it seemed to me that there was just one way forward.

Just as there are mouse embryonic stem cells, there are human embryonic stem cells. Dr. James Thomson at the University of Wisconsin–Madison and Dr. John Gearhart at John Hopkins University independently reported the derivation of human embryonic stem cells from embryos (made by in vitro fertilization) and from fetuses (after abortions), respectively, in 1998. Just like mouse embryonic stem cells, the human version could also be grown indefinitely in dishes in the laboratory. A researcher could start with a single stem cell and over the course of a few weeks turn it into billions of stem cells.

The human embryonic stem cells were also pluripotent, meaning they could be turned into any of the adult body's cell types. Over the next decade, researchers worked out procedures to convert the stem cells into nerve cells, heart muscle cells, liver cells, vascular cells, and other cell types in the laboratory. This meant that researchers could now grow and study as many, say, vascular cells as they wanted without worrying about having to obtain them directly from human beings.

Yet research using human embryonic stem cells became quite controversial due to the origins of the cells from human embryos or fetuses. For those who sincerely believed that human embryos are life rather than potential life—the same as live-born babies, children, and adults, and deserving of the same dignity and respect—the destruction of human embryos to make stem cells was tantamount to murder. Since 1995, the U.S. Congress has passed the Dickey–Wicker Amendment to appropriations bills every year. It forbids the use of federal funds for "the creation of a human embryo or embryos for research purposes" or for "research in which a human embryo or embryos are destroyed, discarded, or knowingly subjected to risk of injury or death …" Yet the Amendment doesn't forbid the use of federal funds for research using human embryonic stem cells after they have already been made, which was confirmed by rulings from U.S. federal courts in the early 2010s.

On August 9, 2001, U.S. President George W. Bush announced that he was signing an executive order that permitted federal funding of research using human embryonic stem cells already made prior to that date. (He cited stem cells made from sixty embryos.) At the same time, the order banned federal funding of research using any new human embryonic stem cells made from that date forward. He viewed his executive order as a thoughtful, carefully crafted compromise balancing the concerns of those who viewed human embryos as life and those who saw great promise for new medical treatments and relief of human suffering through stem cell research. Reportedly he saw his decision as one of the most consequential he'd make as President. (This was a month before the 9/11 terrorist attacks.)

Unfortunately, most of the human embryonic stem cells made prior to August 2001 were of poor quality, not suitable for use in research. Stem cell scientists found themselves in the peculiar position of having to make new human embryonic stem cells and doing research with those cells in their laboratories, but not being able to use federal funding for any of that research. This forced them to use non-federal funding (state funding, private foundation funding, philanthropy) to buy equipment, chemicals, and laboratory supplies. Some researchers furnished whole rooms that were explicitly set aside for human embryonic stem cell research. It got to the point where even a pack of test tubes would have to be labeled with a sticker designating it as permissible for stem cell research. This would ensure that not a single dollar of federal funding was accidentally used to support stem cell research.

Subsequently, majorities in both the U.S. Senate and House of Representatives twice passed legislation to permit the use of federal funding to support research using any human embryonic stem cells made from embryos that otherwise would have been discarded (made by in vitro fertilization but ultimately not used for pregnancy)—as long as the funding didn't support the actual act of creating the stem cells from embryos, in line with the Dickey–Wicker Amendment. President Bush vetoed the legislation both times. This state of affairs was resolved only after the election of President Barack Obama in 2008. In 2009, he issued an executive order rescinding President Bush's executive order of 2001. While he couldn't overturn the Dickey–Wicker Amendment, he did considerably loosen restrictions on stem cell research.

Ironically, scientific advancements had already rendered President Obama's action largely moot. In 2006, Dr. Shinya Yamanaka at Kyoto University in Japan reported that he could convert or reprogram adult mouse cells into pluripotent stem cells by inserting just four genes into the cells. These four genes became known as the Yamanaka factors, and the cells became known as induced pluripotent stem cells, or iPSCs. By the end of 2007, several research teams including Yamanaka's team showed that the same factors could also turn adult human cells into induced pluripotent stem cells. It now was possible to take a small sample of skin cells from an adult, or even cells from a routine blood draw, and turn them into induced pluripotent stem cells. Because these cells didn't involve embryos at all, the federal funding restrictions didn't apply.

Although there initially were concerns that the induced pluripotent stem cells weren't of the same quality as human embryonic stem cells, that ultimately proved not to be the case. By the early 2010s, it was no longer necessary for researchers to use human embryonic stem cells and, in doing so, have to bend over backward to adhere to restrictions on federal funding. In part to recognize the importance of induced pluripotent stem cells for biomedical research, the Nobel Prize in Physiology or Medicine was awarded to Yamanaka in 2012.

In 2008, as I was pondering how to study new genetic factors involved in heart disease, I settled on human embryonic stem cells and induced pluripotent stem cells as the best strategy. These cells checked off all of the necessary criteria. They had human genomes. They could grow indefinitely, meaning I could expand them into billions of cells as needed. They were pluripotent, so I could coax them into becoming vascular cells, heart muscle cells, or liver cells. Best of all, they were amenable to genetic modification. Capecchi and Smithies had figured out how to get homologous recombination to work in mouse embryonic stem cells. After Thomson and Gearhart had established human embryonic stem cells, various researchers had attempted homologous recombination in the cells. And it worked, although it didn't seem to work as efficiently as it did in mouse cells. So in principle I'd be able to produce large numbers of genetically modified adult-type cells and study heart disease in a dish.

I started working in the laboratory of Dr. Chad Cowan, a stem cell scientist at Massachusetts General Hospital, to master the husbandry of human embryonic stem cells. They were finicky cells that required constant attention. I had to feed them every single day (even weekends) with a fresh mix of nutrients, and also make sure that they didn't overgrow on the dish. Otherwise they had an unfortunate tendency to spontaneously turn into adult-type cells. They'd no longer be stem cells—and I'd have to start all over again.

After learning how to care for these cells, I started to experiment with homologous recombination. One of the first things I tried was to snip out a small part of chromosome 9 that had recently been linked to heart disease. This turned out to be an arduous task. Even using the antibiotic tricks developed by Capecchi and Smithies, modifying the genome was very inefficient. I ended up having to examine many hundreds of cells to find just a single one with the desired deletion.

Worse, in working with the cells I had to put them through a lot of manipulations: removing them from one dish; soaking the cells in a solution filled with synthetic DNA molecules intended to drive homologous recombination; zapping the cells with an electric current to temporarily open up holes in their surfaces and allow the synthetic DNA to flow into the cells; replating the cells in another dish and giving them time to recover; hitting the cells hard with antibiotics and killing off almost all of them; removing and replating the surviving cells a few more times to grow them back to a large number; zapping the cells with electricity a second time to stuff in more DNA molecules; and removing and replating the cells a few more times. It was just too much stress on the cells. By the time I'd found one genetically modified cell and grown it up into a plateful of cells, I could tell just looking at them under the microscope that they'd morphed into something very different from their original form. I was fairly certain this had nothing to do with deleting a tiny piece of chromosome 9. I tried to nurture the cells along to get them to recover, but they petered out and eventually stopped growing altogether. Several months of intensive work down the drain. I went through the whole process again a few times, with no better luck. It was disheartening.

In July 2009, just as I was getting ready to throw in the towel on trying to get homologous recombination to work in human embryonic stem cells, an alliance of three researchers—Dr. Matthew Porteus at University of

Texas Southwestern Medical Center, Dr. J. Keith Joung at Massachusetts General Hospital, and Dr. Linzhao Cheng at Johns Hopkins University School of Medicine—published a paper in the scientific journal *Cell Stem Cell* that caught my attention. They'd been able to improve the efficiency of homologous recombination in human embryonic stem cells and induced pluripotent stem cells by two hundred-fold to fourteen hundred-fold using special proteins called zinc-finger nucleases, or ZFNs. I obsessively pored over the paper to understand the fine details of the work. I came away convinced that ZFNs were going to rescue me.

In all of my attempts at homologous recombination, I was depending on the synthetic DNA sequence pairing up with the native DNA sequence present in one of the cell's chromosomes, due to the two DNA sequences being very closely matched—the only mismatches would be the changes I wanted to flip into the chromosome. But just having the sequences being close to each other wasn't enough to allow the flipping to occur. In order for homologous recombination to happen, there would need to be a physical break in the chromosome within the native DNA sequence. It was the obligatory first step of the process. The cell would then use homologous recombination to repair the break in the chromosome. It would use the synthetic DNA as the template for the repair process, copying over its sequence into the chromosome. The cell would be fooled into copying the mismatches too, planting them permanently into the cell's genome.

The problem with this scheme—the reason the efficiency was so poor—was the need for that initial break in the chromosome. Such DNA breaks happen spontaneously, but very rarely. This is why homologous recombination typically occurred in only one in a million cells.

Porteus, Joung, and Cheng didn't want to rely on a DNA break spontaneously occurring in the right place at the right time by dumb luck. They took matters into their own hands. Their ZFNs were designed to cut DNA. When they zapped their human stem cells with electricity, they made sure the ZFNs got into the cells along with the synthetic DNA molecules.

They used the ZFNs to make a DNA break at exactly the right place in the genome and jump-start the process of homologous recombination. This dramatically boosted the efficiency to unheard-of levels. The modifications they were able to make in the genomes of the human stem cells were quite impressive, and the ZFNs didn't seem to cause any untoward side effects in the cells.

What are these miraculous ZFNs, I wondered, and how did they come to be?

As is the case with most scientific advances, the development of ZFNs involved painstaking work by numerous talented researchers. There are too many to fairly acknowledge in the brief history told here, but it's important to appreciate that all of these researchers, collectively, were responsible for the birth of gene editing.

Sir Aaron Klug at the Medical Research Council Laboratory of Molecular Biology in Cambridge, England, published the first description of zinc fingers in 1985. Klug had received the Nobel Prize in Chemistry three years earlier for the development of an imaging technique called crystallographic electron microscopy. He'd used it to study the structures of DNA and RNA molecules attached to proteins. In the 1985 paper, he reported that a certain protein attached to a certain DNA sequence had multiple similar-looking stretches of about thirty amino acids, occurring over and over again in the protein. Reasoning that these stretches were important for attaching to DNA, he proposed that each stretch of amino acids folded around a zinc atom to form a finger that the protein would stick into the DNA double helix. Particular amino acids in each finger would fit only with specific DNA base pairs, so the protein could use its set of fingers to grab onto one specific DNA sequence. It wouldn't be able to grab onto any other DNA sequences.

In 1991, Dr. Carl Pabo at Johns Hopkins University School of Medicine reported the use of a technique called X-ray crystallography to show exactly how zinc fingers attached to DNA. He found that each zinc finger recognized a specific sequence of three DNA base pairs. An array of three consecutive zinc fingers, then, recognized a full nine DNA base pairs in a row. In his paper, he held out the possibility that it might be possible to identify existing zinc fingers or create new zinc fingers that could recognize any of the sixty-four possible sequences of three consecutive DNA base pairs (four x four x four). If so, zinc fingers might be mixed and matched to create a synthetic protein that could attach to any desired DNA sequence of any desired length, as long as it was a multiple of three base pairs. In 1994, after moving to the Massachusetts Institute of Technology, Pabo reported a technique that allowed his team to custom-build zinc fingers that could grab onto a desired three-base pair sequence—an important step toward building the full library of zinc fingers for all sixty-four sequences.

Around the same time, several other researchers, including Klug, reported similar techniques to build new zinc fingers. Klug used his technique to build a protein with three zinc fingers that together attached to a specific nine-base pair sequence in a cancer-causing gene. Upon inserting the protein into cells, he found that the protein searched through the entire genome and grabbed onto the target sequence in the gene. The protein physically blocked the transcription machinery from converting the DNA sequence of the gene into messenger RNA. This resulted in silencing the gene and inhibition of cancer-like growth of the cells. Several years later, in 1998, Dr. Carlos F. Barbas III at the Scripps Research Institute in La Jolla, California, was able to assemble a protein with six zinc fingers that together attached to an eighteen-base pair sequence in a different cancer-causing gene and blocked its transcription.

At around the same time, Dr. Srinivasan Chandrasegaran at John Hopkins University was studying a bacterial enzyme called *Fok* I. This enzyme had evolved so as to recognize a particular DNA sequence, grab onto it, and cut both DNA strands, causing a full double-strand break in the DNA molecule. In 1993, Chandrasegaran reported that different parts of the *Fok* I enzyme were responsible for the DNA sequence recognition versus the DNA cutting. Aware of the ongoing work with zinc fingers, he set out to create a totally new kind of protein. He fused three zinc fingers to the DNA-cutting portion of the *Fok* I enzyme. He made two of these proteins, each recognizing a different DNA sequence. He found that each of the proteins could cut synthetic versions of the target DNA sequence in test tubes. He reported his work on these two proteins—the very first zinc-finger nucleases (ZFNs)—in 1995.

In parallel with these scientific developments, other researchers were investigating how cells repair double-strand breaks in DNA. Dr. Maria Jasin at the Sloan Kettering Institute in New York City had been working with a yeast enzyme called I-*Sce*I. This enzyme recognizes a specific eighteen-base pair DNA sequence and creates a double-strand break in that sequence. Jasin inserted this specific DNA sequence into the genome of mouse cells. She could then introduce the I-*Sce*I enzyme into the modified cells and cause double-strand breaks in the target sequence, now present within the genome itself. The idea was to add a synthetic DNA matching the sequence around the I-*Sce*I target site, with the hope of causing homologous recombination in some of the cells. When she used I-*Sce*I and the synthetic DNA together, there was a more than one hundred-fold increase in the rate of homologous recombination compared to the use of the synthetic DNA alone. This showed the power of using a DNA-cutting enzyme to introduce the double-strand break to kick-start homologous recombination, rather than hoping the necessary double-strand break would fortuitously happen on its own.

Yet Jasin saw that a second repair mechanism was occurring too. In this mechanism, the cell took the two free ends of DNA generated by the double-strand break and attempted to simply put them back together, without any involvement by any other DNA sequence as a repair template. In scientific parlance, this is known as non-homologous end-joining (NHEJ). Usually this crude attempt at repair worked just fine, and the original sequence was restored as if nothing had happened. But every so often, NHEJ repair resulted in an error. Base pairs would be lost from the rejoined DNA sequence. Exactly how many base pairs were deleted seemed to be random, or at least semi-random (there were some patterns, but they were hard to predict). The deletions were as small as one base pair and as large as fifty-two base pairs. In one case, there was actually an insertion of one extra base pair into the sequence.

Jasin's work showed that homologous recombination and NHEJ were both being used to heal DNA breaks in the genome in the I-*Sce*I-treated cells—competing, side-by-side. She reported this landmark study in the journal *Molecular and Cellular Biology* in 1994.

The convergence of three different lines of work—the discovery of zinc fingers and the creation of zinc finger libraries, the fusing of zinc fingers with the DNA-cutting portion of the *Fok* I enzyme, and an understanding of the outcomes of the cell's attempts to repair double-strand breaks in genomic DNA—ushered in the era of gene editing. Dr. Dana Carroll at the University of Utah was the first to achieve the editing of a native gene in the genome of cells, reported in 2002. These cells were within living fruit flies at the larval (immature worm-like) stage, and the targeted gene influenced the body color. Carroll used custom-made ZFNs to make double-strand DNA breaks in the gene, which were then repaired by NHEJ. The resulting deletions or insertions of base pairs in the DNA sequence in some of the flies were semi-random in size, but they all prevented the gene from working properly and changed the body color.

In 2003, Carroll followed up on that work with a similar study— also in fruit flies, targeting the same gene—that demonstrated homologous recombination when a synthetic DNA matching the gene's sequence was slipped into the cells. Also in 2003, Dr. Matthew Porteus, who had been working with Dr. David Baltimore at the California Institute of Technology and had then moved to University of Texas Southwestern Medical Center, reported gene editing with ZFNs in human cells, though he targeted a foreign sequence that had been inserted into the human genome, rather than targeting a native gene.

The achievement of ZFN editing of a native gene in human cells wasn't reported until 2005. Although Porteus was involved in the work, it was largely driven by a company, Sangamo BioSciences (now Sangamo Therapeutics). Indeed, it was Sangamo's scientists who coined the term editing to describe the ZFN-directed genetic modification in their 2005 paper. Sangamo was founded by Edward Lanphier a decade earlier with the goal of developing zinc finger technology for commercial and therapeutic uses. The company's investment in a versatile ZFN platform had now paid off. But Sangamo's control of intellectual property with respect to ZFNs rubbed many academic researchers the wrong way. Sangamo teamed up with Sigma-Aldrich Corporation, a life science and biotechnology company that sold chemicals and supplies to many laboratories, to provide custom-made ZFNs that could target any desired DNA sequence in just six to eight weeks—at a steep price of $25,000 to $35,000.

A group of academic laboratories responded by forming the Zinc Finger Consortium. Led by Dr. J. Keith Joung at Massachusetts General Hospital and including Dr. Daniel Voytas at Iowa State University and Porteus, among others, the Zinc Finger Consortium published a platform that allowed the rapid production and testing of custom-made ZFNs. The platform was freely available to any interested academic researchers. The hope was to make the assembly of zinc fingers highly modular, like putting Lego blocks together.

But the Consortium ran into a major problem. It turned out that simply taking a series of zinc fingers that recognized consecutive three-base pair DNA sequences and plugging them together often didn't yield working ZFNs. In fact, it failed the vast majority of the time. Zinc fingers weren't so modular after all. Sangamo apparently had solved the problem by developing whole libraries of zinc fingers that could attach to any given three-base pair DNA sequence. This gave them a lot of flexibility in mixing and matching zinc fingers. They simply tested a huge number of combinations of zinc fingers and empirically determined which one worked best.

In 2008, the Zinc Finger Consortium published a new library-based, combinatorial platform called OPEN that they thought could match the performance of Sangamo's proprietary platform. OPEN would allow academic researchers to screen through thousands of possible ZFNs and find the ones with the most activity. Joung, Porteus, and Dr. Linzhao Cheng at Johns Hopkins University School of Medicine used the OPEN platform to create the ZFNs that worked so well in enabling homologous recombination in human stem cells in their *Cell Stem Cell* paper—the paper I was avidly reading in July 2009 and that got me keenly interested in ZFNs.

Part of what had me so excited about the *Cell Stem Cell* paper was that Joung was at Massachusetts General Hospital, the same institution where I was doing my stem cell work. Dr. Chad Cowan, as one of my postdoctoral advisors, got in touch with Joung and arranged a meeting. Joung was very happy to help; not only was he willing to make some ZFNs for me to try out in human embryonic stem cells, he offered to share the OPEN platform so I could get ZFN production up and running for myself.

I was all fired up to give the OPEN platform a try. But I spent the next year trying to make ZFNs and had no success. In contrast, the ZFNs that Joung's team made for me using the OPEN platform worked quite well. As generous as he was, I couldn't depend on Joung's largesse for all of the stem cell projects I was eager to get underway, so I found myself at an impasse once again.

Sheer luck with respect to timing saved me.

Dr. Ulla Bonas had been working on a bacterial species called *Xanthomonas campestris* for a long time. These bacteria cause a disease called bacterial leaf spot in pepper and tomato plants, as well as other botanical diseases. She studied virulence proteins that the bacteria injected directly into plant cells, where the proteins could turn off plant defenses and allow the bacteria to thrive. In 1989, while at the University of California, Berkeley, Bonas discovered that one such protein had multiple similar-looking stretches of thirty-four amino acids, all right next to each other, occurring over and over again in the protein—seventeen-and-a-half times to be exact. (The last stretch had only half of the amino acids.) In fact, the stretches were so strikingly similar that they could be considered seventeen-and-a-half near-identical repeats. Almost all of the variation between the repeats occurred at just two adjacent amino acids, in positions twelve and thirteen of each repeat. Over the next two decades, researchers identified similar proteins—containing the same mysterious repeats—made by other *Xanthomonas* bacterial species.

In 2007, now at Martin Luther University Halle-Wittenberg in Germany, Bonas reported that her original seventeen-and-a-half-repeat protein could attach to DNA, specifically a DNA sequence in a native gene in the plant genome. In doing so, the bacterial protein increased transcription of the gene, acting to turn up the gene's activity. This resulted in enlargement of the plant's cells and other changes that made the plant more vulnerable to the bacterial infection. Now that it was understood that they grabbed onto DNA and activated transcription of plant genes, the virulence proteins became known as transcription activator-like effectors (TAL effectors), and their distinctive repeats known as TAL repeats.

Dr. Adam Bogdanove at Iowa State University had been studying virulence factors produced by *Xanthomonas oryzae*, which infects rice plants, for several years. His work had taken him in the direction of TAL effectors. As additional target DNA sequences of various TAL effectors came out of the woodwork, Bogdanove and Bonas independently realized that there was roughly a one-to-one correspondence between the number of repeats in each TAL effector and the number of base pairs in the DNA sequence recognized by the effector. For example, Bonas' original seventeen-and-a-half-repeat protein from *Xanthomonas campestris* seemed to attach to sequences about eighteen or nineteen base pairs in length. This symmetry allowed the two researchers to break the TAL code. The variable amino acids in positions twelve and thirteen specified the base pair to which that particular TAL repeat attached.

The code was elegant. If the two amino acids were histidine and aspartate (HD), the TAL repeat specified C; if asparagine and isoleucine (NI), it specified A; if asparagine and glycine (NG), it specified T; if asparagine and asparagine (NN), it specified G [later work would show that asparagine and lysine (NK) also specified G]. Asparagine and serine (NS) acted as a wild card—the TAL repeat accommodated any of the four base pairs. Bonas took the TAL code one provocative step further. She created seven artificial TAL effectors using the code and found they could turn on genes that contained the predicted target sequences. Bonas and Bogdanove reported the TAL code in two papers published in the same issue of the journal *Science* in December 2009.

Having been stymied in my efforts to broadly deploy ZFNs in the service of gene editing in human embryonic stem cells, I read Bonas' and Bogdanove's papers with great interest. I realized it might be possible to create new gene editors by fusing an array of TAL repeats, specifying a target DNA sequence, with the DNA-cutting portion of the *Fok* I enzyme. Of course, many other researchers were thinking exactly the same thing. Bogdanove teamed up with Dr. Daniel Voytas, who'd moved from Iowa State University to the University of Minnesota, and created the first TAL effector nucleases (TALEN). They reported their success in July 2010. Over the next year, several groups published similar reports, with a team of scientists at Sangamo showing that their versions of TALENs worked remarkably well in human cells. Guided by Bogdanove's and Voytas' paper, I started creating a platform to build TALENs and deliver them into human embryonic stem cells, building on my prior experience with ZFNs.

All of this was happening around the time I was wrapping up my postdoctoral research fellowship and applying for a faculty position. It was while interviewing at Harvard Medical School that I first met Dr. George

Church. Church is widely known for his pioneering contributions to science (genome sequencing technologies, synthetic biology, and the Personal Genome Project, among many others), his entrepreneurship (co-founder of more than twenty companies), and his provocative proposals (recreating wooly mammoths and, most infamously, Neanderthal humans, though he subsequently made it clear that the latter was just a thought experiment). My conversation with Church centered on my work with human embryonic stem cells, and he endorsed the notion of using TALENs for gene editing of stem cells. His team had been experimenting with TAL effectors, he told me, and they'd found them to be quite pleasant to work with. Church mentioned that the TAL effector work in his laboratory had been spearheaded by a young scientist, Dr. Feng Zhang, who recently had been recruited to a joint faculty position at the Massachusetts Institute of Technology and the Broad Institute. He suggested that I speak to Zhang.

Shortly afterward, I dropped by Zhang's office at the Broad Institute to chat. I filled him in on what I was trying to do with human embryonic stem cells. He was amiable and quite happy to share his TAL effector platform, which he'd be publishing very soon; he even printed out a preliminary version of his paper for me. By the time I met Zhang, I was already halfway done with building my own TALEN platform, but some elements of Zhang's platform would be useful, so I gladly took him up on his offer.

Once I had my TALEN platform up and running, I tested it out with regular human cells. I knew that using TALENs in human embryonic stem cells might be more difficult, so I didn't want to start there. I decided to target a sequence on chromosome 1 that I had recently found to be linked with cholesterol and heart disease. I hedged my bets by building a bunch of TALENs that I predicted would create double-strand breaks at various positions around the target sequence, remembering my travails with ZFNs and thinking that most if not all of the TALENs wouldn't work. I was hoping just one would show some activity. So I was shocked when every single one of the TALENs showed signs of working, and working well! It seemed that TALENs were highly modular, plug-and-play, in a way that

ZFNs were not; it really was like putting Lego blocks together. I understood now why Church had called them pleasant.

A couple of days later, I was at a dinner with several faculty members from the Broad Institute. I was suspicious about the TALENs working so well, and I told Dr. Stuart Schreiber, one of the dinner guests, about my concerns. His response was that I had the right scientific instincts—if something looked too good to be true, it probably wasn't true. But as I continued to work on the TALENs over the next few months, I came to the inescapable conclusion that they really were that good, at least when used in regular human cells.

But Schreiber's advice proved prescient. When I tried to put the same TALENs into human embryonic stem cells, I saw zero activity. I tried again and again. No luck. After a lot of troubleshooting, I realized that the TALENs were too big to easily slip into human embryonic stem cells. (The regular human cells I'd tested had soaked them up with no difficulty.) Even after shocking the stem cells with electricity to temporarily open up holes in their surfaces, very few of the cells were picking up the TALENs.

It took two years of work to figure out how to get TALENs to work in stem cells. By then I had taken my first faculty position at Harvard University, in the new Department of Stem Cell and Regenerative Biology. My laboratory was in a newly renovated building on the college campus, on the same floor as Cowan, my recent postdoctoral advisor, who'd moved his own laboratory from Massachusetts General Hospital to Harvard. Working with Dr. Qiurong Ding, a postdoctoral research fellow being advised jointly by Cowan and me, I devised a scheme by which we were able to coax any stem cells that picked up the TALENs into glowing both green and red. We could then use a fancy and very expensive machine called a fluorescence-activated cell sorter to pick out the glowing cells and discard the non-glowing cells. Conveniently, my new department happened to have a few of these machines just down the hall from us; we could use them at any time of the day or night (and we did).

Now that we had a way to purify the stem cells carrying the TALENs, we could figure out whether the TALENs were any good at gene editing. We started by designing TALENs to target sequences in a few genes linked to heart disease and disorders of metabolism. Our goal was to use NHEJ repair to introduce small deletions or insertions right into the middle of the genes. By trimming away base pairs or stuffing in extra base pairs, we were hoping to create frameshift mutations that would inactivate the proteins coded by the genes. With the first gene we tried, we found that TALENs were able to edit about ten to twenty percent of the stem cells. This was better than we'd ever seen before, even with Joung's ZFNs.

Encouraged by these results, I wanted to build up our TALEN platform so that it would be possible for us—or any other researcher, anywhere—to build TALENs with a single day of work, instead of the weeks of work it had been taking us to make each new set of TALENs from scratch. This meant creating prefabricated blocks with every possible combination of three or four consecutive TAL repeats, 832 in total. We could easily assemble any TALEN for any fifteen-base pair DNA sequence by simply mixing and matching the correct four blocks. It took a huge amount of effort and about a year of time for us to create the full collection of blocks, but the end result was well worth it.

Once we had the final platform ready to go, we were able to make TALENs, get them into stem cells, and edit fifteen different genes in just a few months. Before, I had struggled for years to do just one gene! The efficiency of editing varied widely—anywhere from two percent of the cells to a full third of the cells. But compared to the pre-gene-editing era, even our least efficient TALEN editing was a bonanza. We published our TALEN platform and the results of in-depth studies of four different genes in the journal *Cell Stem Cell* in December 2013. It took more than five years to get to this point, but I'd finally succeeded in realizing my vision of using adult-type cells made from genetically modified stem cells to study heart disease.

Little did I realize it would be just a matter of weeks before much of my work became instantly obsolete.

5

CO-OPTING CRISPR

After the publication of our *Cell Stem Cell* paper, I took a break from research and worked as a physician for two weeks—which just happened to overlap with the winter holidays. When I'd accepted my faculty position at Harvard, I'd also agreed to serve as an attending cardiologist at Brigham and Women's Hospital in Boston a few times a year. This meant I supervised a team of trainee physicians taking care of patients hospitalized for serious heart problems. I welcomed these opportunities to personally help people get through acute medical issues and send them home feeling much better. My time in the hospital provided a nice contrast to toiling away in the laboratory, where it might be decades before my research led to a therapy that would help patients.

Then on January 3, 2013, my world turned upside down. My time on hospital service was coming to an end. I was already thinking ahead to my return to the laboratory, and how to take advantage of our new TALEN platform to make a fresh effort to understand heart disease. But that day, two back-to-back papers were published online by the journal *Science*, one from Dr. Feng Zhang at the Broad Institute and one from Dr. George Church at Harvard Medical School. They reported the successful use in human cells of a new gene editor with a mouthful of a name: clustered regularly interspaced short palindromic repeats (CRISPR)–CRISPR-associated 9 (Cas9).

These papers didn't catch me totally by surprise. I was well aware that CRISPR-Cas9 was under active exploration due to its gene-editing potential. Zhang and I had both contributed to a proposal for a large grant of funding from the U.S. National Institutes of Health that we submitted in January 2012. My contribution was my laboratory's expertise with genetics, TALENs, and human embryonic stem cells. Zhang's contribution was a proposal to use the CRISPR-Cas9 system to develop a new gene editor. Zhang hadn't included any preliminary data showing his success yet, but it was clear that his laboratory was aggressively working on CRISPR-Cas9.

The existence of CRISPR was first noted by Dr. Atsuo Nakata of Osaka University in Japan in 1987. While studying an unrelated protein in the bacterial species *Escherichia coli*, he noted the existence of a cluster of five repeat sequences that were each twenty-nine base pairs in length, separated by variable sequences, or spacers, with a fixed length of thirty-two base pairs, in the bacterial genome. He subsequently found the same repeat sequences in the genomes of other bacterial species, but he didn't take the work any further.

A few years later, Dr. Francisco Mojica at the University of Alicante in Spain noticed similar repeat and spacer sequences in a different group of microbes and, investigating further, reported in 2000 that they were present in at least twenty different species. These unusual DNA sequences were soon found to be associated with a set of nearby genes and received the name CRISPR. Over the next few years, Mojica studied the spacer sequences between the repeat sequences. He eventually realized that they matched up with sequences in the DNA molecules of viruses that infected the bacterial species. He proposed that CRISPR was an immune system that somehow stored in the bacterial genomic DNA a record of past viral infections and, presumably, could use that recorded information to fight off future repeat infections by the same viruses.

The notion of CRISPR as an immune system was confirmed by Drs. Rodolphe Barrangou and Philippe Horvath at Danisco, a food company, in elegant work that was published in 2007. They showed that a protein coded by one of the nearby CRISPR-associated (Cas) genes was necessary for bacteria to fight off infections by viruses whose sequences were recorded in the CRISPR system. This protein later came to be known as Cas9. Other Cas proteins were involved in capturing sequences from invading viruses and copying them into the bacterial genome as spacers.

The following year, Drs. Luciano Marraffini and Erik Sontheimer at Northwestern University proved that the CRISPR-Cas9 system worked by cutting DNA molecules rather than RNA molecules. Moreover, the DNA did not need to be from invading viruses; CRISPR-Cas9 would destroy any piece of double-strand DNA with a matching sequence. Dr. Emmanuelle Charpentier at Umeå University in Sweden, working with Dr. Jörg Vogel at the University of Würzburg in Germany, provided a crucial piece of the puzzle in discovering that the bacterial CRISPR-Cas9 system utilized two RNA molecules—an RNA transcribed from a spacer sequence plus a repeat sequence (already known as the CRISPR RNA or crRNA) and a separate, novel RNA called the tracrRNA. They reported this work in 2011.

Charpentier then teamed up with Dr. Jennifer Doudna at the University of California, Berkeley, to take the three components of the system—the Cas9 protein, the crRNA, and the tracrRNA—and see if they were sufficient to cut DNA in test tubes. The answer was yes. They then showed that if they changed the portion of the crRNA that corresponded to the spacer sequence—the first twenty bases—they could reprogram the system to cut a double-strand DNA molecule with the new sequence of twenty bases. Finally, they cleverly fused the two RNA molecules into a single RNA molecule, a so-called guide RNA, and turned a three-component system into a two-component system. This simple system worked, too. So they now had a new programmable gene editor that worked in test tubes.

Doudna and Charpentier submitted a manuscript describing their work to the journal *Science* on June 8, 2012; it was published online June 28, 2012, a remarkably short time later. The editors at *Science* clearly understood the importance of the work. Doudna's long-standing reputation as a brilliant researcher surely didn't hurt, either.

Dr. Virginijus Šikšnys at Vilnius University in Lithuania was simultaneously pursuing the same goal of recreating the CRISPR-Cas9 system in a test tube. With the help of Barrangou and Horvath, he succeeded—possibly earlier than Doudna and Charpentier. Šikšnys submitted his manuscript to the journal *Cell* in April 2012. Inexplicably, the editors of *Cell* immediately rejected it without subjecting it to peer review. (If a submitted manuscript is deemed of interest by journal editors, it's sent to independent researchers with expertise in the topic of the manuscript. As peer reviewers, the researchers judge whether the paper should be accepted, revised by the authors after doing more studies, or rejected. Very rarely do peer reviewers recommend immediate acceptance. Editors can choose not to send a manuscript for peer review at all if they feel it's not suitable for the journal.) Šikšnys then submitted the manuscript to the journal *Proceedings of the National Academy of Sciences of the United States of America* on May 21, 2012. It was published online September 4, two months after Doudna's and Charpentier's *Science* paper.

That *Science* paper captured a lot of people's interest, including my own. It seemed like there was a reasonable chance that this new gene editor would work in human cells. It could be as simple as putting Cas9 and a guide RNA into cells and seeing if it caused editing in the human genome. I was briefly tempted to give it a try myself. But I figured that with people like Doudna and Zhang and who knows how many other people pursuing the exact same goal, if there were anything to it, it would be solved soon enough. (Zhang's and Church's papers would be published just six months later.) I was perfectly happy to be an early adopter of new technology; no need for me to be the one developing the technology unless it was absolutely necessary. My interest here was to be able to do gene editing in stem cells, and by the summer of 2012 my laboratory was getting great results with TALENs.

Zhang and Church weren't the only researchers who'd successfully implemented CRISPR-Cas9 as a gene editor in human cells as of January 2013. Within a few weeks of their back-to-back *Science* papers being published online on January 3, Doudna published her own report in the journal *eLife*, and Dr. Jin-Soo Kim at Seoul National University in South Korea published a report in the journal *Nature Biotechnology*. Back-to-back with Kim's paper, Dr. J. Keith Joung of Massachusetts General Hospital published a report in *Nature Biotechnology* in which he successfully implemented CRISPR-Cas9 in fish.

Out of these five papers, the first had been submitted for publication on October 5, 2012, and the last had been submitted on December 18, 2012. For purposes of scientific credit, it really should be regarded as a five-way tie for first place. It is also clear that all five papers drew inspiration from Doudna's and Charpentier's June 2012 *Science* paper; all of them included some version of the guide RNA made from a fusion of the tracrRNA and the crRNA. But timing is everything. Because of their lead of just a few weeks, Zhang's and Church's papers are the ones that have received the most attention and that most researchers cite as the foundational CRISPR-Cas9 gene-editing papers.

I was at the nurse's station on 10 West in the Shapiro Pavilion at Brigham and Women's Hospital when I learned about Zhang's and Church's papers. I printed them out immediately and gave them a careful read. Fortunately, my medical team had no patients who were particularly sick—they all were convalescing nicely—and it was a quiet afternoon, so there was no guilt in putting aside my medical duties for a little while. Still, it must have been a strange sight: I had the various pages of the two papers spread over every available space on the main table at the nurse's station.

Upon reading the papers, I came away with the impression that Church's implementation of the two-component CRISPR-Cas9 system was working somewhat better than Zhang's. So I had one of the students in my laboratory reach out to Church to see if he would be willing to share his CRISPR-Cas9 system with us. He was. By the time I finished up my two-week stint of hospital service and was back in the laboratory, we had Church's system in hand and were ready to start working with it.

The big question on my mind was whether CRISPR-Cas9 had much to offer. Sure, it looked like it could do gene editing, but there were already well-established gene editors—ZFNs and TALENs. CRISPR-Cas9 seemed pretty easy to use. To redirect CRISPR-Cas9 to a different site in the genome, one only needed to change the first twenty bases in the guide RNA, which could be done with a single day of work in the laboratory. But we had already built a TALEN platform that would allow anybody to make new TALENs with a single day of work. So CRISPR-Cas9 would only be useful if it worked as well as or better than TALENs. Based on the data in Zhang's and Church's papers, it wasn't clear that was the case.

I realized my laboratory was uniquely positioned to do a head-to-head comparison of TALENs versus CRISPR-Cas9. We had already developed a platform to deliver TALENs into human embryonic stem cells. We had also already used TALENs to successfully edit more than fifteen genes in stem cells. And we had already cataloged the efficiencies of the TALENs for all of those target sequences in the human genome. So why not swap out the TALENs and swap in CRISPR-Cas9 and see how well the latter worked at some of those same target sequences? I huddled with Dr. Qiurong Ding, the postdoctoral fellow in my laboratory who had the most familiarity with the TALEN platform, and we hatched a scheme to quickly put CRISPR-Cas9 through its paces.

It ended up being pure grunt work. I designed and engineered each CRISPR guide RNA and handed it off to Ding. She used an electric charge to push the guide RNA and Cas9 into stem cells, sorted out the glowing cells that had received CRISPR-Cas9, and then laboriously isolated and grew hundreds of individual cells for analysis. She purified genomic DNA from the cells and used PCR and Sanger sequencing to evaluate the CRISPR-Cas9 target site. I then pored over the chromatograms and determined how often edits were occurring. We set up a pipeline so that we could test many different target sites in quick succession. It was a miserable month for Ding and me, working around the clock. But we pressed on.

On a day in late February 2013, we got our first sense of whether CRISPR-Cas9 was working well. Ding was analyzing a full batch of PCRs. She was doing quality control, assessing whether the PCR-amplified sequences were the correct size, before sending the samples for Sanger sequencing. This involved looking at about one hundred samples in a single picture. Ding came over to my desk and said, in a deceptively understated way, "it looks like CRISPR works."

That immediately got my full and undivided attention. I dropped what I was doing and ran over with Ding to look at the computer monitor showing the picture. And what I saw stunned me. So many of the PCR samples looked like they had DNAs that weren't the right size. What I instantly realized was that most of the sequences had deletions or insertions that were throwing off their sizes. The conclusion was inescapable and electrifying—not only did CRISPR-Cas9 work for gene editing in human stem cells, it worked like gangbusters.

Over the next couple of weeks, the data poured in. They were unbelievable. At eight target sites we'd tested with TALENs, the efficiencies had ranged from none of the cells being edited to thirty-four percent of the cells being edited. (We made sure to include the one case we found where TALENs failed altogether.) There was a lot of variability, but that's how it was with TALENs—some worked really well, some not so well. At the same eight target sites, including the one with zero TALEN activity, CRIS-PR-Cas9 resulted in efficiencies ranging from fifty-one percent of the cells being edited to seventy-nine percent of the cells being edited. The worst CRISPR-Cas9 editing worked far better than the best TALEN editing! It wasn't even close.

Even before all of the data had come in, I knew we'd made a crucial observation. We had unequivocal evidence that CRISPR-Cas9 was vastly superior to previous gene editors. Combining that with how easy it was to use, CRISPR-Cas9 had all of the advantages. It was going to make gene editing accessible to everyone, not just specialist researchers.

I wrote to Dr. Deborah Sweet, who at the time was the editor-in-chief of the journal *Cell Stem Cell*. I had communicated with her when getting our TALEN paper published in that journal just a couple of months earlier. I gave her a quick rundown of our results, explaining how much better CRISPR-Cas9 was performing compared to TALENs. She wrote back almost immediately expressing her interest, but not quite sure whether it made for a substantial enough story to warrant publication. But then I heard from her again, just hours later. She'd had the chance to review the data more closely and think about them further during her spin class. She realized just how dramatic the results were, and she suggested that I write up the work as a Letter to the Editor. That way she could expedite the processing of the manuscript and, if all went smoothly with the peer review process, the journal could publish it in the next month's issue.

Following Sweet's advice, Ding and I wrote up the manuscript and submitted it to the journal within a few days. I framed it as a follow-up note to the TALEN paper from December, now showing that CRISPR-Cas9 outperformed TALENs across the board. Writing the manuscript was a bittersweet experience. Effectively I was conceding that all of the work we had done with TALENs was now obsolete and should be ignored, and that everyone should start using CRISPR-Cas9 instead. At least, I thought, it was us making our own work obsolete. It would have been so much more painful if somebody else had made our work obsolete.

The manuscript sailed through peer review, and true to her word, Sweet included it in the April 4, 2013, print issue of *Cell Stem Cell*. From the day Ding and I started our work with CRISPR-Cas9 to the day the letter was published was a mere ten weeks.

After the publication of the letter, my laboratory never used TALENs again.

In its simplest implementation, the CRISPR-Cas9 gene editor has just two components: the Cas9 protein and a guide RNA about one hundred bases in length. One protein and one RNA assemble into a unit, a molecular machine that scans across any double-strand DNA molecule with which it comes in contact. If placed into the nucleus of a human cell, the machine will scan across all forty-six chromosomes of the human genome. It pauses whenever it comes across a short DNA sequence known as a PAM. It then takes the first twenty bases of the guide RNA and tests to see if the base sequence matches the DNA base pair sequence at that location. If there's a perfect match (or, sometimes, a near-perfect match), the machine will clamp down on the DNA molecule and cut both strands. The machine then moves on.

The key to CRISPR-Cas9 as a gene editor, then, are those first twenty bases of the guide RNA (known as the protospacer sequence). Think of CRISPR-Cas9 as having a built-in GPS navigator. Changing just those twenty bases is the same as putting a new address into the GPS and sending the machine to a different location in the genome.

CRISPR-Cas9 is often compared to the search-and-replace feature in a word processor. But that's not a good way to portray it, as it grossly oversimplifies what's happening. Instead, imagine the human genome as a book, with each chromosome a different chapter, and each gene a sentence.

CRISPR-Cas9 makes a double-strand break in the DNA at the site where a change is wanted. This is like ripping the page so that the tear goes right through the word that needs to be edited. There are two options for repairing the double-strand break, NHEJ and homologous recombination. (Researchers often refer to the latter by the alternative term homology-directed repair, abbreviated as HDR). NHEJ repair is like simply taping the page up. Sometimes the original language remains perfectly clear. But if the pieces aren't taped back together exactly right, or if some of the letters are lost because of the roughness of the tear, the word or sentence won't read the same after the page is taped up. This is great if deliberately trying to inactivate a gene, trying to garble a certain word or sentence on that page in that book.

Homologous recombination is like fixing a torn page by ripping that entire page out of the book and taping back in a freshly printed version of the page. In this scenario, if the goal is to correct a typo in a word on a page, then the replacement page would need to have the correct spelling of the word. This process is a lot more complicated than a search-and-replace, which would involve simply erasing the offending letter and writing in the correct one. It's part of the reason why homologous recombination is so inefficient. But search-and-replace simply isn't an available option when using CRISPR-Cas9.

Though there was no mention of it in our *Cell Stem Cell* letter, the thought had occurred to me: *if CRISPR-Cas9 works so well in human embryonic stem cells, and human embryonic stem cells are very similar to the cells in human embryos, then … CRISPR-Cas9 should work really well in human embryos, no?* Not that I had the slightest interest in answering that question, but someone was bound to make the same connection and act on it.

In no time at all, researchers were exploring how well CRISPR-Cas9 worked in embryos—mouse embryos, that is. Zhang had teamed up with

Dr. Rudolf Jaenisch at the Whitehead Institute for Biomedical Research, affiliated with the Massachusetts Institute of Technology, to explore whether CRISPR-Cas9 could speed up the process of making knockout and knock-in mice. The answer was a resounding yes. In a paper published in May 2013, they reported that when they injected CRISPR-Cas9 directly into mouse zygotes made by in vitro fertilization, it efficiently knocked out genes via the introduction of frameshift mutations by NHEJ repair. Once the resulting embryos were transferred into mothers, mice with full gene knockout were born after three weeks of pregnancy.

Though it didn't work as efficiently as it did for gene knockout, if CRISPR-Cas9 was injected along with a synthetic DNA sequence into mouse zygotes, it could edit specific changes into genes by homologous recombination in some of the zygotes. Again, this could yield knock-in mice in just three weeks.

Drs. Martin Evans, Mario Capecchi, and Oliver Smithies had received the Nobel Prize six years earlier for developing methods to make knockout and knock-in mice with mouse embryonic stem cells, and the whole process of making the mice took one to two years. Now, seemingly overnight, CRISPR-Cas9 had reduced the time to less than a month and dispensed with embryonic stem cells altogether.

Researchers immediately started to test out CRISPR-Cas9 in zygotes of other animals. They had widespread success—indeed, there didn't seem to be any animal for which the technique didn't work. This culminated in a team of Chinese scientists, led by Drs. Xingxu Huang, Weizhi Ji, and Jiahao Sha, using CRISPR-Cas9 in zygotes to make genetically modified monkeys, which they reported in early 2014. In evolutionary terms, monkeys are humans' close cousins. So when I read the Chinese team's paper, it confirmed my already-strong conviction that CRISPR-Cas9 would work quite well in human zygotes, and that we'd all better start thinking very seriously about the prospect of gene-edited babies.

Just three months after the Chinese team's paper was published, Drs. Canquan Zhou and Junjiu Huang at Sun Yat-Sen University in Guangzhou, China, injected CRISPR-Cas9 into human zygotes. They used zygotes that had been rejected by fertility clinics as being non-viable—meaning there was no chance of a successful pregnancy, and thus no possibility of gene-edited babies. They targeted a gene called *HBB*, which codes for a portion of the hemoglobin molecule that ferries oxygen in the bloodstream. Mutations in *HBB* can cause either sickle cell disease or another blood disorder called beta-thalassemia. Zhou and Huang found that CRISPR-Cas9 edited the *HBB* gene in more than half of the human embryos. They also found they could use a synthetic DNA sequence to get homologous recombination to occur, successfully inserting mutations into *HBB* in a small proportion of the embryos. This raised the likelihood that a future attempt would be made to correct disease-causing *HBB* mutations in human zygotes. Indeed, the researchers' choice of a disease gene as the one to target in this first study seemed to broadcast an intention to eventually move toward gene-edited babies.

Ominously, the embryos showed signs of potentially dangerous side effects from CRISPR-Cas9—so-called off-target effects. The CRISPR-Cas9 unit was intended to make a double-strand break in a target sequence in the genome, pointed to the right location by the GPS-like guide RNA. More specifically, the first twenty bases of the guide RNA. What if the matching twenty-base pair DNA sequence at the target site wasn't the only place in the genome where that twenty-base pair DNA sequence occurred? Put another way, what if the address 3000 Walnut Street was put into a GPS, and there was a 3000 Walnut Street not only in the intended town, but also in another nearby town? It might very well end up going to the wrong place. With CRISPR-Cas9, this would mean going to another location in the genome, making a double-strand break, and potentially causing an unintended mutation.

This might not be a problem if the address 3000 Walnut Street only exists in the one town. But what if there's a similar-sounding address—3000

Walnut Avenue or 3000 Walnut Lane—in the next town over? Unless paying close attention, it might still be possible to end up in the wrong place. CRISPR-Cas9 doesn't always require a perfect match between the first twenty bases of the guide RNA and the DNA molecule it's scanning. It's a bit promiscuous. If it finds a DNA sequence with one, two, or even three or more mismatches with the guide RNA, it might occasionally make a double-strand break there. Why is this a big deal? Imagine if the use of CRISPR-Cas9 in a human embryo inadvertently caused a mutation in a gene that's linked to cancer. It's possible that a person born from that embryo would be at greatly increased risk of cancer in her lifetime. If CRISPR-Cas9 happened to hit exactly the wrong gene, it could mean childhood cancer or even multiple childhood cancers. Or it might cause some other grievous disease.

Zhou and Huang looked for off-target effects in their CRISPR-Cas9–treated human embryos. They focused specifically on locations in the genome that had sequences that might confuse CRISPR-Cas9 by their similarity to the desired target site in *HBB*. And they found unintended mutations in a large proportion of the embryos. They acknowledged this serious safety issue in the final sentence of their manuscript describing the work: "In particular, off-target effect of CRISPR/Cas9 should be investigated thoroughly before any clinical application."

From a technical perspective, the work of Zhou and Huang wasn't much of an advance. All of the results were in line with what one would have predicted in light of past studies with embryos from different animal species, including the off-target effects. But the fact that these were human embryos added a whole new dimension to the story, one that was decidedly non-scientific. Zhou and Huang submitted the manuscript about their work to the most prestigious scientific journals in the world, *Nature* and *Science*. The manuscript was rejected by both journals, at least partly due to ethical objections raised by the reviewers. Word got out about the manuscript, and prominent scientists immediately started calling for a moratorium on any gene editing of human embryos. Zhou and Huang ultimately ended up publishing their work in an obscure journal in China in April 2015. Nonetheless, the publication captured worldwide attention, unleashed a storm of controversy, and inspired a spate of magazine covers with pictures of imagined designer babies.

Yet the notion of a moratorium didn't end up carrying much weight. A number of Chinese researchers followed up on Zhou's and Huang's work, testing out CRISPR-Cas9 on various disease genes in non-viable embryos and then viable embryos. The work wasn't limited to China, though. In a study published in September 2017, Dr. Kathy Niakin at the Francis Crick Institute in London knocked out a gene called *POU5F1* in viable human zygotes and found this to impair the development of the resulting embryos. What distinguished Niakin's study from those of the various Chinese researchers were two things. First, her study was explicitly couched as basic research aimed at gaining scientific knowledge, at understanding the process of early human development in the womb. There wasn't the slightest hint of an ambition to eventually make gene-edited babies. All of the embryos were destroyed within seven days after fertilization. Second, she applied for and received formal regulatory approval from the appropriate government agency, the U.K. Human Fertilisation and Embryology Authority. Everything about her study was transparent and above board.

In contrast with Niakin, Dr. Shoukhrat Mitalipov at Oregon Health & Science University very much had gene-edited babies on his mind. He recruited a patient with a serious inherited heart disease called hypertrophic cardiomyopathy, in which the heart muscle is thickened and prone to life-threatening abnormal rhythms. Found to have a specific disease-causing mutation in the *MYBPC3* gene, the patient donated sperm cells for in vitro fertilization of egg cells from healthy donor women. Because of the genetics of the disease, about half of his sperm cells had the mutation. Mitalipov's team injected CRISPR-Cas9 and a synthetic DNA with the normal *MYBPC3* sequence into the zygotes. In some of the resulting embryos, it appeared that homologous recombination had occurred and corrected the mutant *MYBPC3* gene from the patient. (Afterward, there was a protracted scientific debate about whether precise gene editing had actually occurred and, if so, the mechanism by which it occurred.)

In theory, the gene-corrected embryos could have been implanted into the womb of a mother, who after nine months could have given birth to children who would be free of the father's disease. What actually happened is that Mitalipov's team exhaustively dissected the embryos to study how the desired edits had occurred and whether there were off-target effects from CRISPR-Cas9. Any remaining embryos were destroyed within two weeks after fertilization.

Since Mitalipov's embryo research was performed in the United States, the Dickey–Wicker amendment being passed each year by Congress prevented federal funding of the work. Instead his team relied on private funding. There's no U.S. federal agency equivalent to the U.K. Human Fertilisation and Embryology Authority. So Mitalipov's institution, Oregon Health & Science University, created an extensive regulatory framework to ensure the research was done in an ethical manner. It took Mitalipov two years to receive approval for the study. When finally published in August 2017, Mitalipov's work raised little public controversy compared to Zhou's and Huang's paper two years earlier. (This was in spite of news about Mitalipov's paper leaking a week before its actual publication.) In interviews, Mitalipov was quoted as saying that it would be five to ten years before gene editing of embryos would be ready for use to prevent disease in babies.

By the autumn of 2017, it was abundantly clear that human embryo editing could be done—indeed, already had been done many times by many researchers—and that there were no scientific barriers to taking gene-edited embryos through pregnancy to live birth. The only thing that had prevented the world's first gene-edited baby from being born was that no researcher had been willing to cross that line.

6

BETTER HEALTH THROUGH GENE EDITING?

As a cardiologist, patients are never far from my mind. So when I realized how astonishingly well CRISPR-Cas9 worked in human embryonic stem cells in February 2013, my thoughts turned immediately to the possibility of using CRISPR-Cas9 as therapy. I'd been thinking for years about genetic superheroes with inactivating mutations in *PCSK9* or *ANGPTL3*. It was a very short leap to think about using CRISPR-Cas9 to put those same mutations into regular folks and protect them against heart disease.

With Dr. Qiurong Ding and I generating loads of impressive data with CRISPR-Cas9, it quickly came to the attention of my colleagues at Harvard. Drs. Chad Cowan and Derrick Rossi, the latter an expert in bone marrow stem cells, immediately wanted to try to target *CCR5* in both bone marrow stem cells and T cells. HIV therapy was on their minds. We teamed up to get some experiments done over the next few months. It soon became clear that CRISPR-Cas9 could edit *CCR5* by means of NHEJ repair in both cell types, though not as efficiently as in human embryonic stem cells.

In parallel, I thought it'd be worth spending some effort to explore whether CRISPR-Cas9 could address sickle cell disease, a horrific disease that affects both kids and adults. It occurs most commonly in populations in sub-Saharan Africa and people with ancestors from that part of the world. It's caused by having two copies of a particular missense mutation in the *HBB* gene that causes its coded protein, a subunit of hemoglobin, to have the amino acid valine in the sixth position instead of the amino acid glutamate. Hemoglobin's role is to carry oxygen in red blood cells, delivering it to all of the tissues of the body. The mutation causes the protein to become sticky and to aggregate into long chains that distort the red blood cell into a sickle-like shape. These sickle cells are fragile and prone to breakage, which reduces the oxygen supply to the body.

The sickle cells also tend to get trapped in small blood vessels. Occasionally this problem escalates in severity, causing a crisis in which blood flow to downstream tissues is blocked. A variety of organs can sustain damage during a crisis. But perhaps the worst feature of a crisis is the pain—excruciating, debilitating pain that can last for days and is difficult to treat. During my medical training I'd taken care of a number of sickle cell disease patients while they were hospitalized in the throes of a crisis. They experienced suffering I have yet to see surpassed by any other group of patients.

Because there's only one mutation that causes sickle cell disease, it would make developing a gene-editing strategy more straightforward. In contrast to other diseases that are each caused by a variety of different mutations, working out how to correct the one *HBB* mutation would mean being able to treat all sickle cell patients. On the flip side, correcting the mutation would require homologous recombination. It would be a more difficult proposition than using NHEJ repair to insert inactivating mutations into a gene like *CCR5*.

We obtained induced pluripotent stem cells, made from a patient with sickle cell disease, from Dr. George Daley's laboratory at Harvard Medical School. We then slipped CRISPR-Cas9 along with a synthetic DNA with the correct *HBB* sequence into the cells. Our hope was that we could correct the missense mutation in at least one of the two defective copies of the *HBB* gene. Correcting just one copy in a patient's cells would be enough to cure the disease, since carriers of one normal copy and one mutant copy are healthy. (In fact, there's evidence that carriers of one mutant copy are protected against malaria. This might explain how the mutation came to be so common in sub-Saharan Africa, where malaria is prevalent.)

In our pilot experiment, we screened several dozen CRISPR-Cas9–treated cells. One cell had a single corrected copy of the *HBB* gene. Not the most efficient outcome, but it made for a nice proof of concept, and we now were in a position to grow disease-free stem cells matched to a sickle cell disease patient. Though not feasible with today's technology, in the future it might be possible to use those stem cells to make bone marrow that could be transplanted back into that patient and permanently cure the disease.

Even before getting these early signs of success with *CCR5* and *HBB*, we'd started to give serious thought to starting a company. Rossi had recently co-founded the company Moderna, which uses RNA molecules as vaccines. Through that experience, he knew people at various biotechnology-oriented venture capital firms in the Boston area whom we could approach. But the first step was to pay a visit to Dr. George Church at Harvard Medical School. He'd co-founded many companies in his career. More importantly, he was one of the several researchers who'd more-or-less simultaneously published the first uses of CRISPR-Cas9 in human cells. He'd kindly shared his version of the CRISPR-Cas9 system with my laboratory in January, and it was the same version we had working so well in stem cells. I'd emailed Church to let him know about the impressive efficiency of CRISPR-Cas9, but it'd be good to fill him in on the full results in person.

In early April, Rossi and I went over to Church's laboratory to meet him. After filling him in on the latest data—which duly impressed him—we asked whether he'd be open to working with us to approach venture capital firms and try to raise interest in starting a company. Church said yes, he'd be quite interested in that.

So started a spring of Church, Cowan, Rossi, and I making the rounds with various venture capital firms in the Boston area. Given Church's and Rossi's track records at starting successful biotechnology companies, all of the firms were interested in speaking with us. By the time we met with them, each of them had already heard whispers about CRISPR-Cas9. But our team was uniquely capable of filling them in on the full details of the technology and some of the therapeutic opportunities. Each time we pitched our proposal, the scene-stealer was my presentation of the head-to-head comparison of CRISPR-Cas9 versus TALENs—the worst CRISPR-Cas9 targeting being far better than the best TALEN targeting. That really got the message across that this wasn't just another gene editor. CRISPR-Cas9 was a game-changer.

Not a single firm we met with failed to be excited about the possibility of funding a startup company around CRISPR-Cas9. But the situation was complicated. Several other pioneers in the CRISPR-Cas9 arena had also started exploring the commercial potential of the technology: Drs. Feng Zhang, J. Keith Joung, Emmanuelle Charpentier, Jennifer Doudna, and others. Church advised reaching out to the others and seeing if there was interest in teaming up. And that's how, years after first meeting her when I was in graduate school, I got to meet Doudna again.

As a graduate student at The Rockefeller University in the late 1990s and early 2000s, I worked in the laboratories of two mentors: Dr. Robert Darnell, an RNA biologist and neurologist, and Dr. Stephen Burley, a structural biologist. I focused on proteins whose purpose seemed to be interacting with certain messenger RNAs in cells in the brain and spinal cord, where they had a role in neurodegenerative disease. I wanted to understand how each protein directly interacted with each RNA molecule. Put another way, what parts of the protein reached out and grabbed onto what parts of the RNA strand? I set out to answer this question by producing and purifying large quantities of various pieces of the protein and the RNA. I then mixed protein and RNA together and attempted to grow crystals of the combined components. The idea was to fire powerful X-rays at the crystals, capture the images resulting from the shadows cast by the protein and RNA, and use the data from the images to reconstruct a full molecular portrait of the juxtaposed protein and RNA—a process known as X-ray crystallography.

This was tedious stuff that required a lot of troubleshooting, and it took years to bring it to successful completion. Naturally, in the process of doing this project, I looked to the published work of other researchers who had tackled similar projects. I was hoping to pick up tips that could speed up my own efforts. And that's how I first came to know about Dr. Jennifer Doudna, who years later would become a pivotal figure in the story of CRISPR.

At the time, Doudna had a reputation among my circle of colleagues as being an enormously talented crystallographer and a rising star in RNA biology. After completing her graduate and postdoctoral training, she started her own research laboratory at Yale University in 1994. She achieved early success by using X-ray crystallography to determine the structure of an RNA molecule that could act as an enzyme and had the ability to cleave itself. It was the largest RNA whose structure had been solved to date, with a sequence 160 bases in length. (By way of comparison, the RNA on which I was working had just twenty bases.) It was a bravura accomplishment that built on five years of her hard work on that particular project.

But what really caught my attention was a paper she published a couple of years later, in 1998. She had been attempting to crystallize another large self-cleaving RNA molecule. Large RNA molecules are typically difficult to crystallize; for a variety of reasons, they don't readily form up into a repetitive, ordered configuration, which is needed to create a high-quality crystal. She found a solution to this problem by finding a way to attach a protein to the RNA. Starting with the original RNA molecule, she was able to build in an extra set of bases into the sequence that didn't interfere with the RNA's normal function. She chose those bases because it was already known they could strongly attach to a specific protein. This well-studied protein had nothing at all to do with the self-cleaving RNA she was investigating, but the extra RNA bases created a bridge between the two molecules.

Past research had found that proteins form crystals more easily than RNAs. This proved to be the case once again. Doudna was able to use the protein to form high-quality crystals, carrying the RNA along with it into the crystals. She was then able to use X-rays to discern the structure of both the protein, which had already been solved by other researchers years earlier, and the self-cleaving RNA—which was entirely novel.

When I first read Doudna's paper in the journal *Nature* reporting this work, I was gobsmacked. Her strategy of affixing the protein as a means of tricking the RNA into forming into crystals struck me as fiendishly clever, a sign of true genius. From that point on I was a fanboy, keeping track of her new publications and poring over the minute details. So I was excited when a couple of years later I learned that Doudna would be visiting Rockefeller to give a scientific talk on her work. I knew that visiting speakers would usually agree to have lunch with a group of graduate students, and I maneuvered to make sure I was on the guest list.

The day came, and it was a thrill to have the opportunity to meet Doudna in person. I didn't get the chance to spend much time with her one-on-one—just a few minutes as I walked with her from her last morning meeting to lunch with the other students. She was very friendly and approachable, but I was daunted to meet one of my scientific heroes and stumbled through a brief description of my own RNA project. Still, lunch provided a nice opportunity to pepper her with questions about her work, and to hear her perspective on being a scientist. Her stellar talk later that day to the Rockefeller community only reinforced my impressions of her ingenuity.

Fast forward more than a decade to 2013. Even though I hadn't worked on RNA in a long time, Doudna was still firmly ensconced in my pantheon of scientific heroes. I followed her many accomplishments in the RNA field, and it wasn't at all surprising to me that she'd ended up being pivotal to the development of CRISPR-Cas9 as a gene editor—which, after all, was based on RNA.

Doudna had agreed to make the trip from California to Boston for a couple of days in early June to meet with Church, Cowan, Rossi, and me to talk about CRISPR-Cas9 therapeutics. We convened in my department's building on the Harvard University college campus in Cambridge. I had the chance to chat with her one-on-one in my office. This was a thrilling opportunity to meet with Doudna—not as peers, exactly, but at least as a senior and junior colleague—and show her the data my laboratory had generated. I first ran through the work comparing CRISPR-Cas9 to TALENs in human embryonic stem cells. The data had been published a couple of months earlier, so I was sure she was already aware of it.

Then I showed Doudna something I hadn't shared with anyone else yet, since I had put the pictures together just the previous night, in anticipation of our meeting. It was a set of Sanger sequencing chromatograms showing we had genetically corrected induced pluripotent stem cells from a patient with sickle cell disease. I got the sense that she was quite excited to see this real-world demonstration of the therapeutic potential of CRISPR-Cas9.

After Doudna had the chance to meet with the others one-on-one, we went out to lunch in Harvard Square. We heard a firsthand account of how she and her postdoctoral fellow, Dr. Martin Jinek, had turned the naturally occurring bacterial three-component CRISPR-Cas9 system into a streamlined two-component system. They were meeting in her office, discussing the finer points of the structures of the crRNA and tracrRNA molecules, and had a flash of inspiration that it might be possible to combine the two RNAs into a single RNA. Jinek immediately tested it out in the laboratory and, lo and behold, it worked. This was the genesis of the guide RNA that all practitioners of CRISPR-Cas9 gene editing have been using ever since.

Over the rest of the two days were a variety of meetings we'd set up with Boston-area venture capital firms to introduce Doudna to them. At the end of her visit, we convened again on the Harvard University campus to talk about a potential way forward for a new gene-editing company. It was at that meeting that Doudna made what I thought was a very sensible proposal. She thought that all of the key people who'd made pivotal contributions to CRISPR-Cas9 gene editing over the past year should pool together their foundational intellectual property into a single holding company, which would then in turn license the rights to whatever companies wished to develop CRISPR-Cas9 for commercial applications. One of those companies could be the one we'd been discussing, wholly focused on developing new therapies for diseases like sickle cell disease.

In an ideal world, that's what should have happened. But it's not what ended up happening. As spring turned to summer and I sat in on additional meetings with venture capital firms—at some point or another I was in the same room with each of the researchers who could stake a claim to intellectual property around CRISPR-Cas9—I could sense that tensions had emerged between some of the researchers. In some cases, the disagreements seemed to be about proper attribution of scientific credit. There was already starting to be buzz in scientific circles about a future Nobel Prize for CRISPR-Cas9. In other cases, they seemed to be about financial concerns, personal stakes in a commercial space that was looking to be worth billions of dollars. No doubt the fact that every venture capital firm we'd approached was looking to invest didn't help. There was actually too much money to go around, too much for any single company to soak up. Every investor had come around to the point of view that CRISPR-Cas9 was the scientific breakthrough of the decade, perhaps the century—and they all wanted a piece of the action.

The outcome: three different companies focused on therapeutic CRISPR-Cas9 gene editing came into being by early 2014. The community of CRISPR-Cas9 researchers had been neatly divvied up among the companies as scientific founders and stakeholders. Editas Medicine had

Church, Zhang, and Joung. Intellia Therapeutics had Doudna and Rossi, as well as several long-time stalwarts in the field, Drs. Rodolphe Barrangou, Luciano Marraffini, and Eric Sontheimer. CRISPR Therapeutics had Charpentier, Cowan, and Dr. Matthew Porteus, the ZFN pioneer.

I ended up staying on the sidelines and choosing not to become involved with any of the companies. There were a few reasons. First, I was alarmed by the personality clashes that had emerged among a group of scientific colleagues whom I'd personally found to all be congenial and reasonable people. I didn't like what the distorting influences of scientific credit and financial gain had evidently wrought. Second, I didn't feel I qualified as a CRISPR pioneer—I was a fast follower, at best—or that I merited any sort of financial reward for my work. Third, I wasn't comfortable with what seemed to be a growing irrational exuberance around CRISPR-Cas9 therapeutics. So far, the gene editor seemed to work quite well in cells in a dish, but there was no evidence yet that it worked in a living mammal such as a mouse, much less a human being. Yet hundreds of millions of U.S. dollars were being poured into the companies.

Finally, in my discussions with the companies, I wasn't able to get any of them interested in what I cared about most deeply—coronary artery disease. Sure, they paid lip service to heart disease, but it was clear that it was way down on the list of priorities. The companies' lead programs were based on orphan diseases, rare disorders for which there were no existing treatments, which was laudable and certainly made sense from a business perspective. Orphan diseases offered a fast track to drug approval with the U.S. Food and Drug Administration, as well as the opportunity to command a small but lucrative market for each disease. But that wasn't my passion. I wanted to go after heart disease, the number one killer in the world.

With multiple companies now jockeying for position in the same space, the intellectual property situation became complicated. To many observers' surprise, the Broad Institute was quickly awarded a foundational CRISPR-Cas9 patent by the U.S. Patent and Trademark Office, with Zhang as inventor. What wasn't surprising was that the patent was immediately contested by the University of California, Berkeley, and the University of Vienna on behalf of Doudna and Charpentier as inventors. This led to a long-running legal dispute that seized the scientific community's attention and cast a pall over the gene-editing field. (As of the autumn of 2019, the legal proceedings are ongoing, with no end in sight.) Knowing the principal researchers involved, I wasn't sure what to make of this. Except perhaps the cynical view that a judicial decision concerning a scientific matter, arrived at by a process dominated by non-scientists, was just as likely to get it wrong as it was to get it right.

Some time later I ran into Church, and we reminisced about all the time we'd spent pitching CRISPR-Cas9 to venture capital firms. He was philosophical about the fact that multiple companies had emerged, instead of one. *Probably a good thing, as it means that they'll compete and push each other, which can only be good for the gene-editing field and for the patients who will ultimately benefit from the new treatments.*

I realized that if the companies weren't going to use CRISPR-Cas9 to go after heart disease, I'd have to do it myself. Perhaps if I plugged away at it using the resources of my own laboratory, I could generate data compelling enough to persuade one of the companies to give it a shot.

The obvious gene to start with was *PCSK9*. All of the things that had made *PCSK9* a compelling target for Alnylam Pharmaceuticals when I'd been consulting for them in 2006 were still relevant. With CRISPR-Cas9, there was the possibility of a one-and-done therapy. The strategy was simple: deliver CRISPR-Cas9 into the liver, permanently inactivate the *PCSK9* gene, and watch the LDL cholesterol levels fall for good. There was no need for precise gene editing with homologous recombination. All that was needed was to turn off the gene's activity, any which way. NHEJ repair to put in semi-random deletions and insertions into the gene would do the job nicely. Crude but efficient. It wouldn't even require fully knocking out all the copies of the gene in the liver. People born with a single nonsense mutation in just one of the two copies of the *PCSK9* gene had about a ninety percent reduction in the risk of coronary artery disease. So achieving the equivalent effect with CRISPR-Cas9—editing *PCSK9* with fifty percent efficiency—should be more than enough to benefit patients.

There was only one problem—we had no idea if CRISPR-Cas9 actually worked in the liver. So that was the first question we needed to answer. I once again brainstormed with Ding, the übertalented postdoctoral fellow in my laboratory. We realized that we couldn't just dump CRISPR-Cas9 into a mouse and hope for the best. If that experiment failed and we saw no gene editing, there would be two possible explanations. First, it might be that we didn't get CRISPR-Cas9 into the liver. Second, it might be that CRISPR-Cas9 simply didn't work in the liver. We needed to eliminate the first explanation as an issue so that we could focus on the second. That meant we needed a method that had a one hundred percent guarantee of getting CRISPR-Cas9 into the liver.

The only option at the time was to use a virus. Viruses evolved to infect cells, as it's an essential part of their life cycle. Once a virus gets into a cell, it hijacks the cell's production machinery and redirects it toward making a lot more viruses. Those new viruses then burst out of the cell and go on to infect other cells.

There are two viruses that are routinely grown in the laboratory and that infect the liver very efficiently. The first is adenovirus. The second is adeno-associated virus (AAV). Either virus can be repurposed by researchers to carry genes of their choice into the liver and to use the cells' transcription and translation machinery to make the encoded RNAs and proteins—without reproducing to make more viruses and without killing the liver cells. Researchers generally prefer to use AAV because the body better tolerates it. Adenovirus has an inconvenient tendency to spark a robust antiviral response by the immune system, whereas AAV is able to slip into liver cells unnoticed. But there's a downside to AAV—its cargo size is limited. The standard form of the CRISPR-Cas9 system is too large to fit in AAV. There's no such issue with adenovirus. So Ding and I decided to go ahead with adenovirus. For our purposes, an immune reaction wasn't really a problem, since it wouldn't directly interfere with the process of gene editing in the liver.

We decided to do our pilot experiment with regular mice. It took us a few months to prepare the CRISPR-Cas9 adenovirus, but by the spring of 2014 we were ready to go. Ding administered the adenovirus to several mice through intravenous injections. She waited for three days and then took blood samples and liver samples, with the intent of analyzing them for PCSK9 protein levels and cholesterol levels in the blood and *PCSK9* gene editing in the liver. Doing these analyses took an entire day, and I was at a faculty-student dinner elsewhere on campus while Ding was finishing up the work. I surreptitiously checked my email on my phone over and over again during the dinner, eager to get word from Ding about the results. The suspense was killing me. Finally, after checking my email for about the tenth time that night, a terse message from her: "Well, it worked :)."

Wow, did it ever. The results exceeded my most optimistic expectation. It looked like CRISPR-Cas9 had edited the vast majority of the *PCSK9* gene copies across all the cells of the liver—well above fifty percent. I would have been delighted to see something on the order of ten or twenty percent. The pessimist in me had been sure we wouldn't see anything at all, and that we'd have to do lots of troubleshooting to determine why things hadn't worked. So I was instantly in a celebratory mood, one that was unfortunately lost on the people around me. As the dinner concluded, I walked out across campus with a feeling of triumph.

But when it comes to science, as with so much in life, what one hand giveth, the other taketh away. Just days later, Dr. Daniel Anderson at the Massachusetts Institute of Technology published a paper in the journal

Nature Biotechnology reporting that he'd gotten CRISPR-Cas9 to work in mouse liver. Moreover, he'd been able to use homologous recombination to correct a disease-causing mutation and to cure a fatal disease called hereditary tyrosinemia type 1 (about which there will be more said later in this chapter). A truly impressive result, an experimental treatment resulting in life where before there was only death.

We'd been scooped. It was disappointing not to be the first to report that we'd gotten CRISPR-Cas9 to work in a living mammal. Yet when I read Anderson's paper more carefully, my mood lightened. His team hadn't used a virus to deliver CRISPR-Cas9, but instead had administered pieces of naked DNA into mice with high-pressure injections. Basically just slamming DNA into the liver cells. This didn't typically work too well—only a minority of liver cells would pick up DNA—and this was reflected by the fact that the gene editing occurred at an efficiency of less than one percent. But Anderson's choice to use a mouse model of tyrosinemia was a canny one. Because of the peculiarities of the disease, the effect of genetically correcting even a tiny proportion of cells was greatly amplified, enough to cure the otherwise fatal disease in mice.

From the perspective of gene editing, our own results were turning out to be quite impressive. In repeat experiments, Ding found that the efficiency of gene editing in the mouse liver exceeded fifty percent, the amount of PCSK9 protein in the blood went down by a whopping ninety percent, and the blood cholesterol levels reliably went down thirty-five to forty percent. All of this happened within a few days of the injection of CRISPR-Cas9 adenovirus, and it persisted for weeks. Anderson's paper notwithstanding, we knew our paper would be an important contribution to the scientific literature.

But having been scooped once on this story, I didn't want it to happen again. I was sure there were hordes of researchers doing studies similar to Anderson's and ours. It seemed to me the logical next step in the CRISPR-Cas9 field was to show that it worked in living mammals. So I wanted to get our paper out as soon as possible. Usually it takes more than half a year for a paper to be published, from the time the initial manuscript is submitted, through the entire peer review process, to when it's published in print. Many journals now publish papers online before they appear in the print version of the journal, to speed up things a bit.

Anderson's paper was originally submitted on December 12, 2013, published online on March 30, 2014, and published in print on June 9, 2014. That was actually quite rapid, as papers go. But the premiere scientific journals are notorious for stringing authors along, presumably because they can afford to. For them, it's a buyer's market, with so many researchers vying for the limited space in the journals. Some years ago I had a paper that took more than a year and a half from submission to publication. I have multiple colleagues with papers that took more than two years from submission to publication, and in one case a full five years! I also have colleagues who were strung along by a journal for more than a year and ultimately had their papers rejected—then had to start all over again with another journal.

I didn't want to take the chance of having our manuscript disappear down a black hole at one of the premiere journals. So I decided to go with a specialty journal that publishes research related to heart disease. As I browsed through journal websites, *Circulation Research*, a journal published by the American Heart Association, caught my eye. The journal had a special category of manuscripts for which the editors promised to expedite the peer review process and to make a decision on accepting or rejecting the paper in just seven days. And if the paper was accepted, it'd be published online within twenty-four hours.

Perfect, I thought. Ding and I quickly put together the manuscript and submitted it to *Circulation Research*. Sure enough, in less than a week, we got the decision from the journal. It wasn't a decision to accept the paper for publication outright, but it was clear the editors were interested in the paper and wanted some additional work. Which we were happy to provide; it took only a few additional weeks. Our paper was published online in early June 2014. (In retrospect, I needn't have been so paranoid about getting the paper out as soon as possible. It'd be a full year before any other researchers published a comparable paper.)

We'd established that CRISPR-Cas9 could work really, really well in mice, to the point where it reduced cholesterol by thirty-five to forty percent. If translated to human beings, that would be similar to taking a cholesterol-lowering statin pill every day for the rest of one's life. It might be possible to get that same therapeutic effect with a single shot of *PCSK9* gene editing. It wouldn't be a vaccination, since it wouldn't involve the immune system, but the concept is similar—a single preventive therapy that would confer enduring and possibly lifelong protection against heart disease.

Such a therapy could be a boon. Many people know that heart disease is the leading cause of death in developed countries like the United States and has been for decades. Fewer people appreciate that heart disease is rapidly becoming the leading cause of death in the rest of the world. In a way, this is a sign of success. It means that the traditional scourge of impoverished countries, infectious diseases, is being addressed to the extent that people are living long enough to suffer from noncommunicable diseases like heart attack and stroke.

But it's not great to be trading one killer for another killer. If we take the view that heart disease is the next big global health threat—and I believe we should—then we need to think hard about the best way to deploy a preventive therapy worldwide. The best models we have for successful prevention and even eradication of global killers are the worldwide vaccination programs of the twentieth century. Could gene editing provide the basis of a worldwide program to tackle heart disease in the twenty-first century?

The first of many, many steps toward that goal was to get a sense of whether CRISPR-Cas9 would work in the human liver. The human and mouse versions of the *PCSK9* gene have differences between their sequences (meaning we'd need to use a different guide RNA), and human liver cells are different from mouse liver cells. The other thing we needed to start thinking about seriously was off-target effects. We could look exhaustively for unintended mutations in the mouse genome, but that information wouldn't be very relevant to what happens in the human genome because of the substantial sequence differences between the two. Our best choice would be to focus our efforts on looking for unintended mutations in cells with a human genome.

The easiest way to test the effects of CRISPR-Cas9 on the human liver would be to experiment on human beings. It would also be flagrantly unethical. So we needed a workaround. We hit upon a way to do this using a humanized mouse model devised by Dr. Markus Grompe at Oregon Health & Science University. The idea was to swap mouse liver cells for human liver cells. Use a chemical to kill a mouse's own liver cells, then transplant human liver cells taken from actual human beings (either from a live patient during surgery or from a recently deceased cadaver) into the mouse. Remarkably, the human liver cells would slip into the spaces left behind by the eliminated mouse liver cells, start multiplying, and repopulate the entire liver. We'd then have mice living with human-derived livers.

Making these humanized mice was no trivial task. I hired a surgeon who painstakingly did the surgery for each mouse and carefully nurtured each one back to full health afterward. It took a full year before we had enough mice to do an experiment with CRISPR-Cas9. By that time, a new postdoctoral fellow had joined my lab at Harvard, Dr. Xiao Wang. Wang soon mastered the nuts and bolts of CRISPR-Cas9 gene editing and prepared an adenovirus that would deliver CRISPR-Cas9 into the now-human liver cells. Once in the cells, CRISPR-Cas9 would edit the human version of *PCSK9* in the human genome of those cells. Or so we hoped.

It worked beautifully. Wang saw about fifty percent editing of the human *PCSK9* gene, and a corresponding reduction in the amount of human PCSK9 protein circulating in each mouse's bloodstream. Wang also did a survey for off-target effects at the sites in the genome that were most similar to the *PCSK9* target site. It was as if a desired destination had the address 3000 Walnut Street and she were looking closely at similar addresses across the country: 3000 Walnut Street, 3000 Walnut Avenue, 3000 Walnut Lane, and so forth. She couldn't detect any mutations occurring at those sites. Our conclusion: it seemed that CRISPR-Cas9 worked efficiently and, at a very cursory level, safely in human liver cells in a living animal.

We realized that the same exact adenovirus could be administered to a human being. It'd almost certainly deliver CRISPR-Cas9 into the liver; CRISPR-Cas9 would almost certainly edit *PCSK9*; and the person would almost certainly experience reduced LDL cholesterol levels. But it would be criminal to actually try it in somebody without exhaustive testing in animals first. The only way to do it ethically—maybe—would be if I injected the adenovirus into myself. If I didn't die from a ferocious immune response to the virus, I could see if my cholesterol level fell.

As twisted as it might sound, there's actually something of a tradition of self-experimentation in medical research. The rationale is that the researcher would know better than anyone else the potential benefits and risks of the procedure, and so would be in the best position to give informed consent to the (self-administered) procedure. Dr. Werner Forssmann performed the very first cardiac catheterization, on himself. It worked, and now millions of people have undergone the procedure. Forssmann was awarded the Nobel Prize in Physiology or Medicine in 1956. Dr. Barry Marshall proved that bacteria cause stomach ulcers—contrary to the conventional wisdom at the time—by drinking a broth of bacteria and showing that the bacteria infected his stomach lining (and made him quite sick, in the process). Now patients with ulcers routinely take antibiotics to eliminate bacteria in the stomach. Marshall received the Nobel Prize in Physiology or Medicine in 2005.

I'm neither audacious nor ambitious enough to ever do an experiment like that on myself. Still, our long-term goal was to be able to administer CRISPR-Cas9 to patients and protect them from heart disease for their lifetimes. There was a long process that we'd need to go through to satisfy regulatory agencies like the U.S. Food and Drug Administration and receive the green light to do clinical trials. The next step of that process was to make the gene editing as safe as possible while we were still testing it in mice. We were still very concerned about off-target effects, certainly. But we were also concerned about the unpredictable nature of NHEJ repair. Most of the time, the semi-random deletions and insertions were quite small—on the order of a few base pairs. But there was accumulating evidence from my laboratory and other laboratories that very large deletions and insertions could occur on occasion, as large as thousands of base pairs, maybe even larger. It wasn't clear that these large mutations would cause any problems. But we couldn't rule out unintended consequences, either.

Around this time, I was recruited to the faculty of the Perelman School of Medicine at the University of Pennsylvania. I moved to Philadelphia in the spring of 2016 and soon thereafter welcomed a new postdoctoral fellow to the laboratory, Dr. Alexandra Chadwick. Chadwick had seen me give a talk about my laboratory's work on therapeutic gene editing of *PCSK9* at a scientific conference, and she was keen to contribute to that effort. Her timing turned out to be perfect. It was right as she was settling in that we learned about a major advance in the gene-editing field. It built on CRISPR-Cas9, but was arguably more of a breakthrough than CRISPR-Cas9 itself—a new technology known as base editing.

Nobody had yet solved the problem of precision gene editing, cleanly replacing one single DNA base pair in the genome with another base pair. Even with CRISPR-Cas9 making a double-strand break in DNA, homologous recombination was too inefficient and required using a synthetic DNA sequence in addition to CRISPR-Cas9. Having the extra DNA component made delivery into the liver or another organ in the body much more complicated. Then there was the problem that cells would often use NHEJ repair instead of homologous recombination, even if there was a synthetic DNA sequence present. Some cells might get the desired precise edit, but other cells would pick up semi-random mutations.

Dr. David Liu, a chemist at Harvard University, devised a clever solution to this problem. He decided to partially disable CRISPR-Cas9 so that the GPS function was intact, but the unit could no longer make double-strand breaks in DNA. To this disabled CRISPR-Cas9 unit, Liu's team attached an extra protein, an enzyme that could chemically modify a cytosine base in a DNA molecule so that it was replaced with a thymine base. In other words, a C-to-T edit. It took several rounds of tinkering to improve the efficiency of this new molecular machine. They eventually got it to the point where it could alter genomic DNA in human cells with more than fifty percent efficiency.

With this so-called cytosine base editor, it was now possible to point to a precise location in the genome and make a C-to-T change without the need for homologous recombination. Indeed, the efficiency was much higher than had ever been possible with homologous recombination. And because the base editor didn't make double-strand breaks, the possibility of NHEJ repair causing undesired mutations was precluded, or at least greatly reduced.

Liu's team then tried to make an adenine base editor in a similar way, with the goal of making A-to-G changes. There was a major obstacle, though—there's no naturally occurring enzyme that makes the desired modification of adenine in DNA molecules. But there's a bacterial enzyme that can modify adenine in RNA molecules. The researchers audaciously set out to evolve a new enzyme out of the bacterial enzyme, one that could act on DNA instead of RNA. They did this by making a whole set of modifications in the bacterial enzyme and seeing if any of the changes inched the enzyme toward DNA activity. Adopting the set of changes that seemed to do the trick, they then went through another round of modifications to see if any inched the enzyme even closer to DNA activity. And so forth.

It took seven rounds of modifications, but Liu's team ultimately created an enzyme that acted on DNA with high efficiency. Upon attaching this novel enzyme to a disabled CRISPR-Cas9 unit, they now had a molecular machine that could be pointed to a precise location in the genome and make an A-to-G edit with greater than fifty percent efficiency in human cells. It was a bravura accomplishment. When I first read Liu's paper in the journal *Nature* reporting the creation of the adenine base editor in 2017, I was utterly blown away. No doubt all of my colleagues in the gene-editing field were too.

Liu had created a whole new mode of gene editing. For decades, gene editing was all about double-strand breaks in DNA. Although the tools changed, progressing from ZFNs to TALENs to CRISPR-Cas9, the fundamental approach remained the same as it was in the 1990s. Base editing entirely upended the paradigm. Now it might be possible to use a base editor to correct a single disease-causing mutation, as long as the correction involved a C-to-T or A-to-G change. Instead of relying on homologous recombination, which is like tearing out a whole page of a book and taping in a freshly printed page that has a typo corrected, one could use base editing to do a true search-and-replace to fix the typo.

Though impressed by the potential therapeutic uses of base editors to correct genetic disorders, Chadwick and I were just as excited about the possibility of using a base editor to introduce a specific nonsense mutation into *PCSK9*. The effects would be the same as with NHEJ repair—turn off the gene's activity and reduce the cholesterol level—but achieved in a cleaner, safer way. We wouldn't have to worry so much about unintentionally large deletions or insertions or other untoward effects resulting from double-strand breaks at the target site. But the question, as always, was whether the new technology would actually work in liver cells in living animals.

Chadwick set out to test base editing in mice in the fall of 2016. She first screened all possible sites in the *PCSK9* gene where the cytosine base editor could potentially introduce a nonsense mutation with a C-to-T edit. Using cells in a dish, she found one site in particular that looked quite promising. The next step was to produce an adenovirus to deliver the base editor into the liver. The base editor was even larger than CRISPR-Cas9—it was, after all, a version of CRISPR-Cas9 with an extra enzyme attached—but could still comfortably fit within the cargo capacity of the adenovirus. She then injected the adenovirus into mice.

I was out-of-town in Palm Beach for a University of Pennsylvania fundraiser when Chadwick was analyzing blood and liver samples from the mice in the pilot experiment. It ended up being a replay of what had happened with Ding a few years earlier when she was testing gene editing in mice for the first time. I was at a dinner with prospective donors, obsessively checking my email to see whether Chadwick had an update for me. Late in the dinner: "(EXCITEMENT!!!!!!!!!!!!!!!!!!!!!!!) The samples are liver samples collected today. O.M.G." In the pictures Chadwick sent me, she saw base editing of the gene with efficiency as high as thirty-five percent, with a thirty percent reduction in cholesterol. Once again, the results exceeded our expectations. (Pessimistic, I'd predicted the base editing wouldn't work at all.) Once again, I was in a triumphant mood—surrounded by people who had no idea why I was so cheery.

When I returned to Philadelphia, Chadwick and I brainstormed about next steps. We decided it was time to go after a second heart disease gene, the one Dr. Sekar Kathiresan and I had identified through our search for genetic superheroes: the *ANGPTL3* gene. Chadwick went through the same process as before, screening all the sites of potential nonsense mutations in the gene. After identifying a good candidate, she made a new adenovirus and administered it to mice. It worked even better than it had for *PCSK9*. She achieved editing of the gene in mouse liver with efficiencies as high as fifty percent. This resulted in substantially reduced cholesterol levels and reduced triglyceride levels—two for the price of one.

Encouraged by our success, we started to think about what it would mean to have a one-shot therapy that would permanently edit *PCSK9* or *ANGPTL3* (or maybe even both) in people. We knew that the therapy wouldn't involve the use of adenovirus—it was too dangerous for use in humans. At around that time, Anderson published a report in which his team delivered the components of CRISPR-Cas9 into the mouse liver using lipid nanoparticles. These particles are microscopic capsules of fat into which drugs can be embedded. After injection into the bloodstream, the particles are avidly swallowed up by liver cells, releasing the drugs into the cells. Anderson had targeted the *PCSK9* gene and shown there was substantial gene editing and reduction of cholesterol, just as we'd seen in all our previous studies. This demonstration that viruses weren't needed to deliver CRISPR-Cas9 to the liver was a key step forward in the process of developing gene-editing therapies.

Looking into the crystal ball, years into the future, we thought about which patients might be the first to receive a *PCSK9* or *ANGPTL3* therapy. Whenever one is testing a new medical therapy in clinical trials, one has to consider the potential benefits and risks. For gene editing, the first patients to be enrolled in the clinical trials would be those with the most to gain and the least to lose. Patients so sick that the therapy could have a profound effect on their lives, whether lifespan or quality of life. Any potential harm would be modest compared to their existing illness.

For heart disease, among the patients at highest risk are those with sky-high LDL cholesterol levels, with the severest forms of familial hyper-cholesterolemia. These patients have so much LDL cholesterol that the standard medications like statins can't come anywhere close to reducing it to a reasonable level. They need to be treated by a procedure called apheresis every one to two weeks, often starting in childhood. This involves being hooked up to a machine for several hours at a time to have the cholesterol cleaned out of the blood. It's similar to the dialysis procedure that patients with terrible kidney disease require to stay alive. There's no choice—without apheresis, the risk of having a fatal heart attack is just too high. It's a heavy burden for an afflicted patient to bear.

Chadwick and I decided to try out *ANGPTL3* gene editing in mice engineered to have the equivalent of severe familial hypercholesterolemia. Their cholesterol levels were through the roof. It was possible that the gene editing would work in the liver but still not make much of a dent in the cholesterol levels. That would be important information to know, as it forecast what we might expect to happen in human patients. Now a pro at doing mouse gene-editing studies, Chadwick did the experiment with the high-cholesterol mice.

We'd gotten used to seeing impressive results, but this study took the cake. With the treatment, the mice had both their cholesterol levels and their triglyceride levels fall more than fifty percent. It was so dramatic that we could tell just by looking at the mice's blood samples. Without treatment, the blood was cloudy, full of cholesterol and fat. With the treatment, the blood was almost transparent. We couldn't help feeling a bit giddy about the prospect of doing the same thing for a patient with severe familial hypercholesterolemia. They, too, could go from cloudy blood to clear blood, with a single shot of gene editing, with the effects good for the lifetime. It would mean never having to go through apheresis again. It might even mean the difference between dying young from a heart attack and getting to see children and grandchildren grow up.

Another important consideration is timing. Heart disease is a chronic process that builds over many years. A person receiving the therapy late in life, exposed to high LDL cholesterol for many decades, wouldn't get as much benefit as a person receiving the therapy early in life. In theory, the earlier the better. Still, it would be hard to argue that patients should be getting a cholesterol-lowering treatment during the first few years of life. But it did lead us to some provocative thinking—might there be some diseases where the best option would be to treat patients shortly after birth? Or maybe even before birth?

I met Dr. William Peranteau for the first time soon after I moved to the University of Pennsylvania. There's a stereotype of surgeons being aloof, arrogant, and overconfident. One common joke about surgeons (most commonly told by non-surgeon physicians, in my experience): "What's the difference between God and a surgeon? God doesn't think He's a surgeon." I have certainly run afoul of surgeons who fit that mold to a tee. It never really bothered me, because I have an enormous amount of respect for the fact that surgeons take people's lives into their hands, quite literally. I'd be worried if they weren't absolutely sure of themselves. But I have known many more surgeons who belied the stereotype. Peranteau was one of those. He immediately struck me as one of the nicest people I have ever met, without in any way giving me reason to doubt he'd be in total control of his operating room.

Peranteau was a pediatric surgeon at Children's Hospital of Philadelphia, one of the premiere hospitals of its kind in the world. It happened to be just across the street from the building in which my new laboratory was located. Peranteau was a specialist in that most unusual of surgeries, operating on a fetus while it's still in the mother's womb. Though performed for the first time in 1981, fetal surgeries are still a rarity, performed only by highly specialized teams at select hospitals. It's only used in situations where the fetus has a severe anatomical problem that, if fixed, greatly improves its chance of surviving and being born as a healthy child. This is because the surgery puts not only the fetus at risk, but also the mother. The surgery is similar to a Cesarean section in that the uterus is opened to provide access to the unborn child, but the fetus stays in place while the problem is fixed. Afterward the uterus is closed and the fetus is allowed to continue growing until it's time to be born.

Besides doing pediatric and fetal surgeries, Peranteau was also running a research laboratory program. His focus was on developing stem cell therapies and genetic therapies that could be delivered into babies diagnosed with severe genetic disorders while still in the womb. Most of his work was in mouse models. He'd perfected a technique by which he could carefully open the uterus of a pregnant mouse, isolate each individual fetus (mice can have up to a dozen offspring per litter), and inject cells into a vein that ran right through the primordial liver. Using this technique, he was starting to explore the feasibility of gene editing in the fetus. When Peranteau heard that I'd been doing experiments with gene editing in the liver, he was eager to team up. Likewise, when I heard he had a method for delivering therapies to the fetal liver, I was keen to collaborate with him.

We made an unusual combination—a physician who mostly took care of elderly people with heart disease, and a surgeon who operated on children, before and after birth. But we'd found common ground, and it ended up being a perfect melding of skills and interests. We quickly made plans to build on Chadwick's experiments to see if we could target *PCSK9* in fetal mice. It was just a matter of pairing Chadwick's adenovirus with Peranteau's technique. We used mice whose pregnancies were at day sixteen, which in human terms would be the equivalent of seven months. The procedures appeared to go without a hitch. But there was no way to know if gene editing had occurred until after the treated babies were born.

After the mice were old enough that Chadwick could analyze liver and blood samples, Peranteau brought them over to my laboratory. Chadwick worked all day, and both Peranteau and I were on hand in the late evening when she was finishing up the analyses. No doubt she was feeling a bit put out by the fact that the two of us were hanging around, looking over her shoulder, peppering her with questions, eagerly awaiting the data, and not contributing anything in the slightest bit useful. She took it in stride. Soon enough, we were all able to look at the data together, and it showed that the fetal gene editing had worked! Not only was there substantial editing in the liver, there was substantially reduced cholesterol in the treated mice.

It was a nice success, but we had no intent of actually doing prenatal editing of *PCSK9* in human beings. We didn't see any reason to treat cholesterol before birth; there was no justifiable reason not to wait until the child was born, even if the child had severe familial hypercholesterolemia. But if we could target *PCSK9* before birth, it meant we could target other liver genes before birth. And some of those genes hold the keys to treating congenital diseases that start to cause damage during the fetal stage of life. One such disease is hereditary tyrosinemia type 1, or HT1.

HT1 results from inactivating mutations in both copies of a gene called *FAH*, which codes for an enzyme involved in the breakdown of the amino acid tyrosine in liver cells. Normally, a series of enzymes take tyrosine through a progression of stepwise changes until what's left are small molecules that are either recycled or excreted from the body. The FAH protein is the last enzyme in the chain. If it's not working properly, the partly metabolized products of tyrosine, which are toxic, end up accumulating in the liver cells and killing them. If untreated, this results in liver failure and death soon after a child with the disease is born.

Until the 1990s, the only treatment was a liver transplant. Then it was discovered that a medication called nitisinone, originally developed as an herbicide, could block one of the first enzymes in the chain. This prevented the toxic molecules from being produced in the first place, sparing the liver. Starting in the 1990s, children diagnosed with HT1 were treated with nitisinone. It's a hard medication to take, twice a day, every day, for the rest of the child's life. Skipping the drug could tip the child into liver failure or cause liver cancer. And the medication doesn't block the enzyme perfectly, so some children develop liver problems anyway.

Peranteau and I brainstormed about ways to use gene editing to cure HT1. Think of the liver cell as a bathtub. Water pours in through an open faucet. The water represents the toxic molecules made from broken-down tyrosine. Usually it's not a problem, because the water flows down the drain, and the bathtub remains mostly empty. In HT1, the drain is blocked.

The water fills up the bathtub and spills out of it. That's a dead liver cell. We realized that the simplest way to fix the problem was to open the drain again. That would involve using gene editing to correct the mutations in the *FAH* gene. But we knew that was going to be challenging, because of the limitations of standard gene editing with homologous recombination. We couldn't come up with a way to use base editing to fix the gene, either.

We then thought about how nitisinone works. It's an attempt to address the problem by blocking the faucet, preventing water from flowing into the tub in the first place. It doesn't work perfectly, and it doesn't work for long; the medication needs to be taken again and again and again, perpetually. But we realized we could use gene editing to turn off the faucet for good. We hit upon the strategy of using base editing to introduce nonsense mutations into the *HPD* gene, which codes for the enzyme blocked by nitisinone.

There was an additional factor that would work in our favor. The liver is an incredibly regenerative organ. In Greek mythology, Prometheus gave humankind the gift of fire. The king of the gods, Zeus, enraged by Prometheus' action, chained him to a rock. His punishment: each day, an eagle would fly in and feed on Prometheus' liver. Each night, his liver would grow back. The next day, the eagle would return and start the cycle again. Clearly the ancient Greeks understood something about the unusual properties of the liver.

With HT1, we didn't need gene editing to correct every single cell in the liver. Any cells that we corrected wouldn't fill up with toxic molecules and would survive. Any cells we didn't correct would fill up, and die. As those uncorrected cells died and left space behind, the corrected cells would multiply and fill up the space. Given enough time, the corrected cells would eventually take over the whole liver. The disease would be cured.

Peranteau set things up so that we'd have healthy mouse mothers pregnant with fetuses carrying the HT1 mutations. We compared three different groups of offspring. The first group received no treatment. They all died from liver failure within three weeks of birth. The second group received nitisinone from the time they were born. This matched up well with what happens with actual HT1 patients; they're typically diagnosed soon after birth and started on nitisinone as soon as possible. These mice survived and grew into adulthood. The third group was treated with gene editing while still in the womb. After they were born, they received no medication. They survived into adulthood, proving we'd cured them of HT1.

But there was a surprise. Not only did the gene-edited mice survive, they thrived. Throughout the first several months of life, the gene-edited mice substantially outgrew the medication-treated mice. This continued well into adulthood. The gene-edited mice were unambiguously healthier. When we looked at the livers of the gene-edited mice, we found that the corrected cells had indeed taken over the whole liver. It was a dramatic demonstration of how treating a disease with a genetic therapy rather than a traditional medicine, and doing it early, even in the womb, could make a big difference for health.

Peranteau and I published our fetal gene editing work in October 2018. It received a fair amount of press coverage. We were careful to draw a parallel with fetal surgery, a well-accepted medical procedure. We emphasized that gene-editing therapy should only be used in cases where a fetus had a grievous genetic disorder and was already suffering damage while still in the womb. Otherwise an attempt at fetal gene editing would pose unacceptable risks to the mother. It struck me as noteworthy that not a single person we spoke with raised any ethical concerns about the prospect of fetal gene editing in human beings.

Gene editing of human embryos, followed by pregnancy and live birth, was an entirely different matter, as we—and the rest of the world—would see just a few weeks later.

7

A LINE IS CROSSED

I first met her in November 2017. Little did I suspect that a year later, that meeting would land me a front-row seat to the biggest medical scandal of the decade.

I was in Anaheim, California. It's best known as the home of Disneyland, but Mickey Mouse wasn't on my agenda. I was a few blocks away at the Anaheim Convention Center to attend the American Heart Association's annual Scientific Sessions. With more than ten thousand heart and stroke doctors, nurses, scientists, and other healthcare professionals in attendance each year, this is the Super Bowl of cardiology. If you have ever been to one of these big conferences, you know what it's like. I found myself threading through the crowded halls, immersed in a carnival atmosphere. In trying to get to an event, I'd have to stop every few hundred feet to say hello to a colleague I hadn't seen since the previous year's meeting and wouldn't see again until the following year's meeting—and then rush off again, until I ran into the next person. After each event, somehow the next event would always end up being all the way at the other end of the convention center. So I was chronically running behind. Often there would be several events I badly wanted to attend scheduled at the same time. I would run around trying to catch part of each one, naturally missing the best parts of each. It made for a hectic four days, morning to night.

One evening, I had the rare chance to stop and catch my breath. I was a newly minted editor of one of the American Heart Association's scientific journals—in my case, a genetics journal. I'd been invited for the first time to an exclusive evening cocktail hour for the journal editors and members of the press. To my relief, there was no other event competing for my attention, and I could focus on my assigned task. The job was simple: meet some reporters and get them excited about genetics and, by extension, my journal.

That turned out to be a tall order. An American Heart Association media relations staffer introduced me to several reporters in succession. Upon being introduced to me, each seemed curious until hearing that I was the genetics journal editor. Each time I tried valiantly to talk up genetics. But I couldn't escape the sad truth that the most buzz worthy news in the cardiology world has nothing to do with genetics. People hungrily eat up the latest reports about the latest greatest diet for your heart health, how to squeeze the most benefit out of the least amount of exercise, and amazing new medications or procedures that will save you from heart attacks or stroke and help you live longer. I certainly can't fault anybody for that—I want to know all of those same things too. But with genetics being a complex, nuanced subject, there were no simple and appealing messages for me to pass along. Each journalist politely listened to me for a short while and then moved on.

Then I was introduced to Marilynn Marchione of the Associated Press. Within a minute of conversation, I could tell she was different. Here was someone fascinated not only with genetics, but also with a subject near and dear to my heart: gene editing. And she clearly knew quite a lot about it. We ended up talking, and talking, and talking … and before I knew it, the end of the hour had come and long passed. The room was empty except for Marchione and me gabbing away. It was the kind of conversation that could have lasted hours, but she and I both had places to be. In fact, I ended up being an hour late to a dinner I'd promised to attend after the cocktail hour.

Afterward, the American Heart Association media relations team relayed to me how much Marchione enjoyed meeting me; how great it was that I connected with the most influential journalist in the room. It wasn't deliberate on my part, of course. I was just happy to have fallen in with someone who seemed to appreciate genetics as much as I did.

In a coincidence of timing, a few days later the Associated Press published an exclusive report authored by Marchione on the first use of gene editing in any person's body. The company Sangamo Therapeutics had received government approval to proceed with a clinical trial to treat a rare genetic disorder called Hunter syndrome. Patients lack an enzyme that's important for breaking down and recycling certain carbohydrate molecules. With nowhere to go, the carbohydrates end up overloading various cells and tissues throughout the body. Starting in early childhood, the disease wreaks havoc in multiple organs: deformities of the head, nose, and tongue; ear infections; enlarged belly; thickening of the heart, airways, liver, and spleen; stiffness of the joints; distinctive skin markings on the arms, legs, and back; in the most severe cases, as the brain succumbs, behavioral disturbances and mental disabilities, and then death by age fifteen.

A new treatment called enzyme replacement therapy had become available for patients with Hunter syndrome in just the last decade. The missing enzyme is produced in a laboratory and then administered into a patient's body via a weekly three-hour intravenous infusion into the bloodstream. The enzyme doesn't get to everywhere it needs to go, especially the brain. But this therapy can relieve symptoms and possibly even prolong a patient's life—at a cost of hundreds of thousands of dollars a year.

Gene editing offered a new strategy: once and done. The idea was to use ZFNs to facilitate the insertion of the gene coding for the missing enzyme into a specific location in the genome in some of the liver cells in the patient's body. The gene-editing tools would be delivered directly to the liver using billions of viruses. This would turn the liver into a factory that would continuously pump out the enzyme into the bloodstream for the remainder of the patient's life. This would be a clever way to have the body provide its own enzyme replacement therapy, even if it didn't cure the disease.

Marchione's report described the first patient to receive the gene-editing therapy in the clinical trial: a 44-year-old man from Phoenix, Arizona. Though he'd already lived for an unusually long time for a patient with Hunter syndrome, he'd suffered through twenty-six surgeries to deal with various problems related to his disease. He wasn't expecting a cure and fully understood that he'd continue to have problems, but he was eager to proceed with the experimental treatment. He held out hope for the possibility of not having to go through tedious weekly intravenous treatments any longer. But more than that, he felt he'd be helping future patients with Hunter syndrome by being an early volunteer. He received the treatment on November 13, 2017, with no complications.

This use of gene editing in a patient was unquestionably a historic first. But because the story didn't involve that magic acronym that had so captured the public's attention—CRISPR—the achievement probably didn't receive as much recognition as it should have. A year later, an additional five patients with Hunter syndrome received the treatment. The latest patients had received a substantially higher dose than the first patients. This is a standard design for an initial clinical trial, where the goal is to establish safety of an experimental treatment, first and foremost. Blood tests from the patients with the highest doses showed signs that the therapy might be working. The ultimate test will be to see whether the patients can entirely stop receiving their weekly enzyme replacement therapy infusions and still do well in the long term.

After sending Marchione a congratulatory note about her report, I didn't speak with her again until almost exactly a year later. Once again,

I was at an American Heart Association's Scientific Sessions, this time in Chicago. Once again, I had to navigate an impossibly packed schedule that had me running from event to event nonstop. And once again, I was invited to a Sunday evening cocktail hour specially arranged for journal editors and reporters.

I showed up late, since I found myself in one of those situations where I had to run all the way across the convention center to make it from one event to another. When I entered the room, a bit out of breath, it was already packed with people. No matter—Marchione immediately saw me and came over to say hello. It was as if the intervening year hadn't happened; we picked up right where we left off, chatting about a variety of hot topics in genetics and gene editing. But soon enough Marchione steered the conversation to something that clearly was on her mind— mosaicism. How does it work, and why is it a big deal?

To answer these questions, one needs to understand the natural process by which a human embryo grows from one cell into many cells and, ultimately, a live offspring. It starts with the very first cell—the zygote—that results from the mating of egg and sperm, the process called fertilization. The egg is a giant cell that dwarfs the sperm. Indeed, they hold the distinction of being the largest and smallest human cells in the body, respectively. A sperm's role is little more than to deliver the father's contribution of DNA into the egg. While the egg serves as the sperm's counterpart in that it contains the mother's contribution of DNA, it also carries a large stockpile of nutrients needed to sustain the embryo during its first week. This is crucial, as the embryo is free-floating in the fallopian tube or the uterus and has no external source of nutrients until it's had the chance to implant into the wall of the uterus. That critical event doesn't occur until at least a week after fertilization. Then the embryo can start to draw nutrients from the mother's body.

What this means is that the embryo doesn't grow in size between the time of fertilization and the time of implantation. While a series of cell divisions do occur, turning one cell into several hundred cells, each successive generation of cells is smaller and smaller. This is true if the embryo is in its natural state, in the mother's body. It's also true if the embryo has been produced by in vitro fertilization, in the test tube, and is maintained with a special mix of chemicals that mimic the natural state, outside of the body.

The first cell division, when the zygote splits into two smaller daughter cells, occurs between twelve and twenty-four hours after fertilization. A second round of cell division, taking the embryo from two cells to four cells, occurs within another day. By the third day after fertilization, the embryo has reached the eight-cell stage. Over the next few days, cell division accelerates greatly. By the fifth or sixth day after fertilization, the embryo contains two to three hundred cells and has become a so-called blastocyst. This is the stage at which the embryo is ready for implantation.

Whenever a single cell divides into two daughter cells, there is an obligation to ensure that each of the daughter cells has the same exact genome as the parent cell. This requires a precise duplication of the DNA content of the parent cell. A complicated dance of numerous proteins and enzymes (collectively known as the replication machinery) ensues: coating the double-strand DNA molecule of each chromosome, unwinding the two strands and holding them apart, and using the original strands as templates to construct new strands that are perfectly matched, or complementary, to the old strands. Each new strand is intertwined with the old strand from which it was derived. Out of this process emerges two double-strand DNA molecules that are identical to the original DNA molecule. Or more properly speaking, forty-six double-strand DNA molecules—twenty-three pairs of chromosomes—that are identical to the originals.

At least that's what's supposed to happen. Errors can occur, albeit rarely. Just how rare is a topic of intense investigation and debate among researchers. But in most situations, it's safe to assume that when a single cell divides into two cells, it distributes identical copies of the original genome of twenty-three chromosome pairs to each of the daughter cells. The daughter cells are genetic duplicates or—to use the scientific term—clones.

If all goes normally when a zygote divides into two cells, the daughter cells are clones of the zygote. When each of the two cells divides in turn into two granddaughter cells, all of the four granddaughter cells are clones of the zygote, and each other. This genetic identicalness should be maintained as the cells in the embryo continue to divide, until there are two to three hundred cells in the blastocyst that emerges about a week after fertilization. If all went as expected, if any one cell of the blastocysts were sampled to determine the sequence of the entire genome in that cell, it would be identical to the genome of each and every other cell in the blastocyst.

When mistakes happen, and the cells in the embryo are not perfectly identical, the embryo is said to be mosaic. Let's consider the simplest scenario, where the zygote divides into two daughter cells and an error occurs. Perhaps the replication machinery made a mistake in one of the two copies of a chromosome. One daughter cell inherits the correct version, the other daughter cell the erroneous version. Or perhaps the replication machinery worked perfectly, and the two daughter cells had identical genomes—but then a cosmic ray from space zapped through the mother's body and just happened to strike at one point in a DNA molecule in one of the daughter cells in the embryo, resulting in a change in the sequence.

In either case, the two daughter cells no longer have identical genomes; they're no longer perfect clones. They have a mismatch.

What does this mean for the embryo? Assume everything else goes perfectly from that point onward. The normal daughter cell will divide into two normal granddaughter cells, which will in turn divide into more cells. So, too, will the altered daughter cell divide into two altered granddaughter cells, and so forth. By the time the embryo has reached the blastocyst stage, roughly half of the cells might be normal, and the other half altered. The entire genomic sequence of any one cell of the blastocyst would be identical to the genomes of half the cells in the blastocyst but have a mismatch with the other half of the cells.

The situation can get even more complicated. Let's say the two daughter cells from the scenario above—one normal, one altered—have both divided. There are now a total of four granddaughter cells in the embryo. If a second error, a cosmic ray, or another DNA-altering event should strike in one of the altered granddaughter cells, the embryo will now be a patchwork of four cells with different states. Two cells are normal, one cell has one mismatch, and the last cell has two mismatches. The resulting blastocyst might have one quarter of its cells with one mismatch, and another quarter with two mismatches. This is fairly complex mosaicism.

Of course, issues could occur even later in the process. What if an embryo is at the eight-cell stage, or sixteen-cell stage, or thirty-two-cell stage, and a mismatch arises? The embryo is now mosaic.

If an embryo is mosaic, then it's quite possible that after the embryo has implanted into the wall of the uterus, has grown into a fetus, and finally has been born as a living person, the person will herself be mosaic. She'd be a patchwork of normal cells and cells with mismatches, or even cells with different numbers of mismatches. It could be that cells in some organs all have mismatches, and cells in other organs are entirely spared. It's also possible that an individual organ might itself be a patchwork of cells, with different proportions of normal versus mismatched cells compared to the next organ. It's impossible to predict what will happen.

I have been using the word mismatches as a way of distinguishing altered cells from normal cells—normal meaning the state of the original single cell, the zygote. But another term that's appropriate in this situation is mutations. This is a particularly apt term if one of the DNA mismatches should happen to fall in the middle of a gene that's linked to disease.

Which leads us to Marchione's second question: why is mosaicism a big deal?

Dr. Euan Ashley, a cardiologist at Stanford University, once told me the story of an infant who had a serious, life-threatening problem just one hour after being born. She had an abnormal heart rhythm called torsades de pointes in which the lower chambers of the heart, the ventricles, suddenly started beating far too quickly. There were entirely out of sync with the other parts of the heart. It's the job of the ventricles to pump blood to the rest of the body. So their beating out of control meant that blood with its precious oxygen and nutrients wasn't being circulated effectively to the brain and other vital organs of the body. Without medical intervention, this can be fatal.

The infant's medical team implanted into her a small device, a defibrillator that could detect when abnormal rhythms were occurring and shock the heart back into normal beating. The child's problems didn't end there, though. By six months of age, her heart had ballooned out in size and was no longer able to pump blood effectively, even when it was beating in a normal rhythm. She ultimately needed a heart transplant to survive.

When the medical team looked at the electrical patterns of the heart using a test called an electrocardiogram, they saw that one of the patterns was far too long. This condition is known as long QT syndrome and predisposes the heart to abnormal rhythms like torsades de pointes. Quite often, this syndrome is due to an inherited gene mutation.

Mystery solved—except that there was no family history of long QT syndrome, and routine genetic testing of the child shortly after her diagnosis had turned up clean. So what was causing her disease? Fortunately, Ashley and his team of researchers were experts in cutting-edge DNA sequencing technologies. They performed genome sequencing using DNA isolated from a blood sample from the child. They then carefully combed through the raw data to look for anything out of the ordinary. What they found was evidence of a mutation in a gene called *SCN5A*, which is known to be responsible for long QT syndrome in many cases of the disorder. But there was something odd. In ordinary circumstances, if a person carries a mutation in one of the two inherited copies of the *SCN5A* gene (either the one from the mother or the one from the father), then applying the sequencing technology would show about a fifty/fifty split between the normal sequence of the gene and the mutant sequence. This is because every cell in the body would carry one normal copy and one mutant copy.

The genome sequencing found that there was more like a seventy-six to twenty-four percent split between the normal sequence and the mutant sequence. This could mean that the mutation was not real, just some noise in the system. Or it could mean that the mutation was real but not present in all of the patient's cells. This prompted Ashley's team to perform additional sequencing using DNA from another blood sample from the child, as well as from saliva samples from her parents. Both of the parents came up entirely negative for the mutation. But the child's repeat analysis found a ninety-three to seven percent split between the normal sequence and the mutant sequence.

By now, Ashley's team suspected what you might be suspecting—mosaicism. If the child was mosaic, then the mutation might show up in some parts of her body but not in others. Being observed at a low level in the blood wouldn't predict whether the mutation was present or absent in other tissue samples. After careful analysis of another blood sample, a urine sample, and a hair sample, the researchers estimated that only four to seven percent of the cells in each of the samples had the mutation. The final question, then, was what was happening in the patient's heart, the source of all her medical problems? Was it possible that one hundred percent of the cells in her heart had the mutation, and that was the reason for her severe condition?

Ashley's team wasn't able to answer this question until the child received a heart transplant. Since she no longer needed her old heart, which had been taken out of her body and was ready for disposal, it was straightforward for the researchers to acquire a couple of samples of the heart tissue and analyze them for the presence of the mutation. Surprisingly, only about three to six percent of the heart cells had the mutation. Somehow, that very small fraction of cells having a harmful mutation was enough to cause full-blown heart disease.

With further detective work, Ashley was able to conclude that the patient's mutation had first arisen in one cell in the blastocyst. It wasn't in either of the parents' genes, or in the original zygote. It was an unhappy accident of nature. But it wasn't unique: using their advanced sequencing methods, Ashley's team subsequently identified three other patients with long QT syndrome who turned out to be mosaic for a harmful mutation. They estimate that one in two thousand patients with long QT syndrome started out as mosaic embryos.

There are several lessons to be learned from Ashley's case. First, in cases of mosaicism, standard genetic testing could easily miss the mutation. Second, even if only a small percentage of cells in the body carry a harmful mutation, there can still be life-threatening disease. Third, it's possible that the reverse might be true—if only some of the cells in the body have a protective mutation that guards against disease, the fact that some of the cells are unprotected could mean that the person is still fully vulnerable to the disease.

All of the preceding discussion about mosaicism presumes that mutations occur in cells in an embryo randomly, as rare accidents of nature. But Marchione was asking me about mosaicism in the middle of a conversation about genetics and gene editing. So I knew that she was specifically curious about how CRISPR-Cas9 might cause mosaicism. CRISPR-Cas9 changes the circumstances entirely, because it's a tool used to deliberately introduce mutations into the genome. That being the case, it would be logical to think that CRISPR-Cas9 might greatly increase the risk of mosaic embryos.

This is not a theoretical risk. High rates of mosaicism with CRISPR-Cas9 have been observed in experiment after experiment with animal embryos, going all the way back to 2013. With mouse embryos, rates can be close to one hundred percent. In Dr. Shoukhrat Mitalipov's 2017 paper in the journal *Nature* describing his team's efforts to correct a disease-causing mutation in human embryos, he devoted an entire section of the paper to addressing the problem of mosaicism. Strikingly, he started the section with an unambiguous declarative sentence: "Mosaicism in gene-targeted human embryos is unacceptable in clinical applications." In other words, mosaic embryos should never be used for pregnancy and live birth. His team devoted a substantial amount of effort trying to find ways to minimize the chance of mosaicism occurring in CRISPR-Cas9-treated embryos.

To understand why gene editing and the problem of mosaicism are so intertwined, one needs to be mindful of three facts about CRISPR-Cas9. First, CRISPR-Cas9 editing doesn't occur instantaneously, but is often delayed in action. This is because CRISPR-Cas9 doesn't actually mutate DNA itself. It creates a double-strand break in the DNA, and mutations can sometimes result from the cell's attempt to repair the break. But quite often the cell accurately repairs the DNA, and the original sequence is restored. CRISPR-Cas9 can then come around for another pass and make a fresh double-strand break; the cell attempts to repair the break yet again. Numerous rounds of break and repair can take place before a mutation finally emerges. This whole process can take a lot of time.

Second, the mutations caused by CRISPR-Cas9 are semi-random in nature. In one case, there might be insertion of one base pair; in another case, deletion of one base pair; in yet another case, deletion of two base pairs; and so forth. There can be much larger insertions or deletions. The consequence is that in a single cell, where there are two copies of a gene,

CRISPR-Cas9 can cause zero mutations, one mutation in one copy of the gene, the same mutation in both copies of the gene, or two different mutations in the two copies of the gene.

Third, after being injected into zygotes, active CRISPR-Cas9 units can stick around for hours to days. Within twelve to twenty-four hours, the zygote has divided into two cells. Keep in mind that the embryo hasn't increased in size; rather, it's just divided down the middle. Some of the CRISPR-Cas9 units end up cordoned off in one of the daughter cells, and the other units end up in the second daughter cell. From that point onward, whatever edits happen in one cell are independent from any that happen in the other cell. It's possible that CRISPR-Cas9 might produce no mutations in the original zygote. Across the two daughter cells, there could then be many possible combinations of edits, ranging from zero to a maximum of four different mutations in the four total copies of the gene. More likely is an intermediate result. For example, one of the daughter cells might have no mutations and the other cell might have a single mutation. As the cells continue to divide, and active CRISPR-Cas9 units are passed along into those descendant cells, the range of possible combinations of mutations across the cells becomes stupendously complex. One way or another, the resulting blastocyst is likely to be a patchwork of edits.

To further complicate matters, CRISPR-Cas9 has the potential to cause off-target effects, edits in other parts of the genome. Just as different on-target mutations can arise in different cells in the embryo, so too can different off-target mutations arise in different cells. So the embryo might become mosaic both for desired edits as well as for undesired, potentially harmful mutations.

It should now be apparent why putting CRISPR-Cas9 into embryos is gambling with a roll of the dice, and why Mitalipov's team was so keen to find ways to minimize mosaicism in the human embryos he was trying to repair with CRISPR-Cas9. The best solution they found was to inject CRIS-PR-Cas9 as early as possible, so that most of the units would break down and be inactive by the time the zygote divided into two cells. In one kind of in vitro fertilization, the sperm is injected directly into the egg cell. Mitalipov's team experimented with co-injecting CRISPR-Cas9 units at the same time as the sperm. This procedure reduced the mosaicism, but it didn't eliminate the problem.

When Marchione asked me about mosaicism, I gave her an impromptu explanation similar in broad strokes to the one I have provided here. I'd never tried to explain mosaicism out loud to anyone before. So I soon got to the point where I was making obscure hand gestures, and then I finally started drawing diagrams on napkins. This attracted the attention of another reporter, and after a while I found myself at a table with the journalists sitting to either side, all of us deeply immersed in genetics. Which is what I was supposed to be doing at the cocktail hour anyway.

Just like the year before, our conversation went way past the allotted hour, and we found ourselves in an empty room. Except this time we stayed so late that a convention center staff member was on hand to kick us out. And so it was on to the next event for me, but the next event was already almost over, so it was on to the event after the one I'd now missed. Before we parted, Marchione mentioned that she wanted to get my thoughts on an unpublished scientific manuscript related to gene editing. I would need to keep the manuscript confidential. I agreed without hesitation, saying that I'm always happy to offer a professional opinion when it comes to genetics.

The notion of being asked to look at a manuscript confidentially before it's published was actually quite a familiar one. It's common practice for journals to make papers available to science reporters before the publication date. This gives the journalists enough time to read and digest the papers, interview the researchers who did the work, and contact scientists not involved with the work to get their independent opinions. They can then write their news pieces and have them ready to be released simultaneously with the papers being published. Everyone involved benefits from the coordinated publicity. The journals grant this privilege under the conditions of a press embargo. The reporters, as well as the scientists they interview, have to keep mum on the content of a paper until the exact time dictated by the journal. Woe to the reporter who breaks the embargo by leaking the news to the world ahead of the agreed-upon time, as that reporter is sure to be stricken from the publisher's approved list.

After I returned home to Philadelphia, Marchione and I traded a few emails. I confirmed my willingness to review the manuscript she'd mentioned. She was expecting to receive the manuscript that coming Sunday and would forward it to me immediately. For good measure, she emphasized again that I needed to keep it absolutely confidential. She also didn't want to tell me anything about the work so as not to prejudice my thoughts about it. I told Marchione that I'd make sure to have some free time on Sunday to read the manuscript.

On Thursday, Marchione reached out to me again, asking if I'd be willing to do a remote video interview with the Associated Press about the work in the manuscript. The following Thursday was Thanksgiving, so we'd have to get it done early in the week. No problem, I told her. We agreed to loop in the University of Pennsylvania media relations team so they could help arrange the use of a recording studio on campus. I reached out to the team and filled them in on what I knew, which wasn't much. All I could tell them was that the manuscript had something to do with gene editing.

Naturally, by this point I was aflame with curiosity. Remembering that Marchione had broken the story a year earlier about the first patient to receive gene-editing therapy directly in the body to treat Hunter syndrome, I thought the manuscript might have something to do with that. Perhaps the clinical trial had been stunningly successful. I started mentally preparing myself to make some laudatory comments about gene-editing technology, how it was starting to fulfill its promise of being a revolutionary new means of tackling disease and easing human suffering, and so forth.

I heard again from Marchione on Sunday afternoon, letting me know that she expected to get the manuscript either Sunday night or Monday morning. Because it was Thanksgiving week, my schedule was pretty light. It wouldn't be a problem for me to spend some time going over the manuscript and then to chat with Marchione about it in as much detail as was helpful.

Sunday night—no word from Marchione.

Early Monday morning, checking my email as soon as I was awake— nothing new. I went into work as usual.

I kept a close eye on my email inbox all day. At 1:09 p.m., a message from Marchione popped up in my inbox with a chime. The promised manuscript was attached. I immediately put aside all of my other work and started reading the manuscript.

I will never forget the moment when I realized what the manuscript was about. My instant, involuntary response: "Goddammit!"

A quick glance at the first page of the manuscript told the story. A scientist in China had been doing gene editing in human embryos. He claimed to have implanted embryos in a prospective mother with the intent of causing a pregnancy. Twin girls had been born a few weeks earlier. The edited gene was *CCR5*.

I was shocked, but not really that surprised. The pessimist in me knew that it was only a matter of time before somebody charged ahead and try to make gene-edited babies. But *CCR5*? Clearly the scientist was going for HIV prevention, which struck me as an entirely frivolous excuse to be doing gene editing of babies, since HIV infection was already quite preventable and treatable. I immediately sensed there were going to be serious ethical issues at play here.

The scientist in question was Dr. He Jiankui, who goes by the nickname JK. (To avoid confusion between the surname He and the masculine pronoun he, I will use JK to refer to Dr. He for the rest of the book.) I had never heard of him or interacted with him in any way—or, more accurately,

I had no memory of having ever interacted with him (which subsequent events revealed to be not quite true).

JK had been enrolling couples in a clinical trial with the stated goal of giving them babies who were resistant to HIV. In fact, he'd registered the trial in the Chinese Clinical Trial Registry on November 8, 2018, just a few weeks earlier, though the start date of the trial was listed as March 7, 2017. That meant the clinical trial was post-registered, rather than pre-registered as is the norm. Post-registration would seem to defeat the whole purpose of having clinical trial registries, which are operated with the intent of offering full transparency to the public. Anybody in the world can access registries online, search through the records, and find trials that might be relevant to them. Was the post-registration an attempt by JK to cover himself after the fact, to make things appear right and proper, now that there apparently had been a successful pregnancy?

It just so happened that the Second International Summit on Human Genome Editing, sponsored by the U.S. National Academy of Sciences, the U.S. National Academy of Medicine, the Royal Society of London, and the Academy of Sciences of Hong Kong, was being held at the University of Hong Kong the following week. Many luminaries of the gene-editing field would be in attendance. It was just a short trip from JK's home city, Shenzhen, and I wondered whether JK would be there too.

When I looked at the Summit program on the Internet, I saw that not only would JK be attending, he was scheduled to give a short talk about his research on embryo editing at the end of one of the Wednesday sessions. I was immediately suspicious that JK might be planning to make the first public announcement about the birth of the gene-edited twins at the Summit, perhaps in his talk.

Steve Jobs, the co-founder and CEO of Apple, was famous for his presentations where he announced the company's latest products. One rhetorical device that became widely regarded as a Steve Jobs trademark was his holding off on unveiling the most exciting news until near the end of his presentation. He'd then introduce it with the words, "One more thing ..." and drive the crowd wild in anticipation. Jobs was also famous for his insistence on draconian secrecy about the company's products before the formal announcement. He'd allow a few journalists to preview the products under strict confidentiality, and they'd agree to hold off on publishing their reviews until after Jobs had made his announcement. It was his version of a scientific journal's press embargo.

Was JK planning to unveil the world's first gene-edited babies with a Steve Jobs-style one-more-thing announcement at the end of his talk? It seemed quite plausible, as it would make for the ultimate publicity coup.

This wasn't just any manuscript Marchione had sent me. Her request for my thoughts on the manuscript had taken on a whole new dimension. The biggest question on my mind: were the gene-edited babies the real deal? Or was this Clonaid all over again?

Sixteen years earlier, an announcement of a cloned human baby had rocked the world. In the waning days of 2002, Dr. Brigitte Boisselier, chief executive of a company called Clonaid, held a press conference in Hollywood, Florida. Boisselier's company had successfully created the first human clone, an infant girl named Eve. She was genetically identical to another human being whose cells had been used to create the embryo that resulted in Eve's birth. Because this came five years after the headline-grabbing publication of the paper describing Dolly the Sheep, the first cloned mammal, Boisselier's claim similarly drew intense media interest. Undoubtedly adding to the public's fascination with the story was Clonaid's connection to the Raëlian movement, a religion that teaches that human life on Earth was artificially created by extraterrestrials through cloning. It also teaches that humans should in turn embrace cloning. The movement's leader, Raël himself, spoke out in support of Eve on national television. In the wake of Boisselier's announcement, there was an immediate backlash from scientists and ethicists decrying the cavalier nature of any attempt at human cloning and the serious safety concerns that went along with it.

Nothing came of it all. Boisselier stated from the outset that independent confirmation of Eve being a human clone would be forthcoming. But no such evidence ever came to light. Clonaid made claims over the next few months that additional cloned babies had been born, but each successive claim was given less and less credence. As more months and then years passed with no further news, the story of Eve came to be widely regarded as a hoax. Nothing more than a bizarre play for attention by the Raëlian Church, albeit one that briefly succeeded.

As if there wasn't enough cause to doubt Clonaid's claims already, another very good reason has emerged. It turns out to be exceedingly difficult to clone higher mammals, for a variety of scientific and technical reasons. It wasn't until 2018 that monkeys were successfully cloned for the first time. The leader of the team of scientists in China who achieved this feat, Dr. Mu-ming Poo at the Chinese Academy of Sciences' Institute of Neuroscience in Shanghai, told the journal *Science*: "I would think society and the general public and governments will not allow extension of this method from nonhuman primates to humans." An unintentionally ironic statement, in light of the events that would unfold in Shenzhen and Hong Kong later in the year.

As soon as I learned JK was claiming to have made gene-edited twins, I looked at JK's laboratory's homepage on the website of the university where he was an associate professor, Southern University of Science and Technology in Shenzhen. A quick scan of his publication list confirmed my initial impression that he wasn't a mover and shaker in the gene-editing field, explaining why I'd never heard of him. None of his recent papers had anything to do with gene editing; they were all about DNA sequencing technologies. Nor did he seem to have any sort of medical background.

I also looked carefully at JK's post-registered clinical trial documentation on the Chinese Clinical Trial Registry website. While some of the language was Chinese, enough was English that I could get a sense of what JK's team had been up to. They'd received approval from the medical ethics committee of Shenzhen HarMoniCare Women & Children's Hospital to proceed with the trial. (Notably, the approval was not from Southern University of Science and Technology, although it was listed as the primary sponsor of the clinical trial.) JK's team was recruiting married couples in which the woman was HIV-negative (never infected with the virus) and the man was HIV-positive (previously infected with the virus), but on effective antiviral therapy, so the virus was undetectable in his blood. Each couple had to be willing and able to go through with in vitro fertilization.

Those criteria set off alarm bells in my head. I was already suspicious of *CCR5* as an appropriate target for embryo gene editing. It didn't make any sense to me that the father had to be HIV-positive, and the mother HIV-negative. What was the point of that? There was going to be zero chance of the father passing the virus to a baby. It might have made more sense if it was instead the mother who was HIV-positive. Then there would be a small but credible risk of the mother passing the virus to a baby during the pregnancy or during childbirth.

Included in the clinical trial documentation on the website was a spreadsheet with data about DNA sequences and DNA variants. There were annotations of "Maternal Blood 12 Weeks," "Maternal Blood 19 Weeks," and "Maternal Blood 24 Weeks," a clue there was a pregnancy in the works. I didn't think much of it at the time, since I already knew of JK's claim that gene-edited babies had been born. But this same spreadsheet would end up playing a crucial role later in the course of events.

Back to JK's manuscript. I read through the entirety of the main text and got a sense of the overall story.

Then I started going through the figures that showed pictures of data. And within seconds, I realized two things.

I was absolutely certain that JK's team had actually made gene-edited babies.

And something had gone very, very wrong.

8

A FORENSIC ANALYSIS OF AN EXPERIMENT GONE WRONG

If you're ever having trouble falling asleep, try reading a scientific paper. They tend to be written in a convoluted style, chock full of technical jargon, and couched in mealy-mouthed language that never quite commits to any conclusion. Part of it is the general culture of science—researchers tend to be skeptical folks and are reluctant to make assertions for which there's not unassailable evidence. Part of it is that understanding the work requires highly specialized knowledge that's not easy to convey in lay terms. And part of it might be that not many scientists were literature majors in college.

On the flip side, if you're a researcher and you come across a paper describing work in an area where you're an expert, maybe even work that directly impacts your own work—that paper will be an engrossing page-turner that you won't be able to put down.

Such was the case with the manuscript describing the efforts by JK's team to make the world's first gene-edited babies, as I read through it.

Perhaps the most important part of any paper—certainly the most visible part—is the title. The title of JK's manuscript: "Birth of Twins After

Genome Editing for HIV Resistance." Getting straight to the point, that title certainly was calculated to capture the reader's undivided attention.

The title was followed by a list of the authors and their affiliations. The authors are supposed to be all of those people, and only those people, who made meaningful contributions to the work. (Though it can be highly open to interpretation who did enough to merit authorship and who didn't.) It looked like most of the authors on this manuscript were people working in JK's laboratory at Southern University of Science and Technology in Shenzhen, as part of his research team. But two authors were exceptions. Hua Bai was listed as being affiliated with BaiHuaLin China People Living With HIV/AIDS Alliance, apparently a patient advocacy organization and not a scientific one. Michael W. Deem, the next-to-last author, was listed as being in the Departments of Bioengineering and Physics & Astronomy, Center for Theoretical Biological Physics, and Graduate Program in Systems, Synthetic, and Physical Biology at Rice University in Houston, Texas. *How did an American scientist get caught up in this business?*, I wondered.

Next came the abstract. This is a short summary of the content of a paper, no more than a few hundred words in length. A well-written abstract is like a movie trailer that gives away the full story, intentionally. The first sentence sets the tone. In this case: "Millions of children are born annually with inherited genetic diseases or infectious diseases acquired from parents." It's not at all unusual for a researcher to try to make the work seem more important by invoking how many people are suffering from the disease under study.

On to the meat of the abstract. "The recently developed CRISPR-Cas9 genome editing technique may provide an efficient and cost-effective therapeutic strategy to cure diseases with a genetic component." This general statement was fairly standard for a paper about therapeutic gene editing. "Genome editing at the embryonic stage has potential to permanently cure disease and confer resistance to pathogenic infections." This statement about embryo editing wasn't so standard—now things were getting interesting.

The next few sentences switched from generalities to the specific details of JK's work. "Here, we report the first birth from human gene editing: twin girls who had undergone *CCR5* gene editing as embryos were born normal and healthy in November 2018." There it was—JK's bid to make history. An interesting point here is that scientific journals typically discourage researchers from making a claim of being the first to do something. It's hard to know for sure that there isn't somebody out there in the world who hasn't already done the same thing and just hasn't gotten around to publishing it yet. In JK's case, though, it was probably a reasonable assertion to make.

"Their father was an HIV carrier." I've already noted the oddity of this fact. Why was it important that the father was HIV-positive, when there was basically no chance of a baby becoming infected with HIV via the father? "We used CRISPR-Cas9 to reproduce a prevalent genetic variant of the *CCR5* gene in fertilized oocytes [egg cells] during in vitro fertilization procedure, with the aim of helping the twins to be born with their own natural protection against HIV infection." That made it crystal clear how JK planned to defend the gene editing of babies as ethically sound—invoking a medical need. He didn't identify the specific "prevalent genetic variant of the *CCR5* gene" here, but plainly he was referring to the Δ32 mutation.

"Genome sequencing during pre-implantation genetic testing and after birth confirmed that the twins' *CCR5* genes were edited successfully and are thus expected to confer either complete or partial HIV resistance." *Okay, it sounded like he had done a lot of work to assess the gene editing in the embryos and, later, the babies. But what was this about "partial HIV resistance"? Did that mean the editing hadn't been totally successful?* "No off-targets, large deletions or pathogenic cancer gene mutations was observed." JK was acknowledging the potential problems of gene editing and had apparently looked out for them.

The last two sentences of the abstract were more upsetting. "We here bring a novel therapy to enable acquired immunity to HIV and to control the HIV epidemic." The words "acquired immunity" struck me as problematic. Acquired means something that's gained through a procedure, like vaccination; it seemed to me that was quite different from the circumstance of being born with mutations. Immunity means the immune system having been stimulated so that it can fight off an infection. Having the Δ32 mutation, even two copies of the mutation, is not the same as having immunity. Maybe the consequence—resistance to HIV infection—is the same, but the use of imprecise language could lead to misunderstandings. But the bigger problem here was the talk of controlling the HIV epidemic. How many babies would have to be edited to control a worldwide epidemic? Millions? JK certainly didn't lack for ambition. "We anticipate that human embryo genome editing will bring new hope to millions of families seeking healthy babies free from inherited or acquired life-threatening diseases." Yes, millions. This was making him sound a bit like a megalomaniac, presenting himself as the savior of millions of babies and their families.

After the abstract came the main text of the manuscript. The first paragraph focused on HIV as a public health problem, rather than a biomedical problem. It cited HIV as a cause of death, but also as a cause of discrimination that negatively impacted people's livelihoods, access to medical care, and educational opportunities. I found it noteworthy that the manuscript didn't at all mention the interventions that already have proven successful in preventing HIV infection: effective antiviral medications, methods to prevent sexual transmission, screening of the blood supply to ensure safe transfusions, and so forth.

The next paragraph pivoted straight to a brief discussion of *CCR5* and the Δ32 mutation. It mentioned the prevalence of the Δ32 mutation in Europeans, the disruption of the protein so that it was no longer present on the cell surface, the resistance to infection by most HIV strains conferred by the presence of two copies of the mutation, and the slowed progression to AIDS by the presence of just one copy of the mutation. This was followed by a mention of CRISPR-Cas9 technology and then: "In the present clinical trial, we edited the *CCR5* gene in fertilized oocytes [egg cells] at the single-cell stage to mimic the natural protective genotype of HIV resistant Northern Europeans … and provide newborns with lifelong protection against HIV infection." From this statement, one might have thought that JK's intent was to exactly reproduce the *CCR5* Δ32 mutation with CRISPR-Cas9 gene editing.

But the next section of JK's manuscript made it clear this wasn't the case. It stated that the CRISPR-Cas9 gene editing targeted the exact start of the Δ32 mutation. But there was no intention to make the precise Δ32 deletion. Instead, the goal was to use NHEJ repair to introduce semi-random frameshift mutations into the same location in the *CCR5* gene as the Δ32 deletion. The rationale was that any frameshift mutations would have the same effect as the Δ32 mutation. But was that in fact a reasonable assumption?

Gene editing that involves making double-strand breaks in DNA—whether by CRISPR-Cas9, TALENs, or ZFNs—has substantial limitations. If the goal is to simply stop a gene from working, NHEJ repair will get the job done. It is crude, but effective. The repair will result in semi-random mutations at the target site. There is no way to control the size of any particular mutation in any particular copy of the gene. But that's okay if any deletion or insertion of DNA base pairs will mess up the coded protein.

If the goal is to make a precise deletion or insertion, things get a lot harder. For the most part, the only way to get this kind of change is through homologous recombination with a synthetic DNA sequence that closely matches the target site but also carries the desired change. The cell might be fooled into copying over the desired change into the target site in the genome. But it's also quite possible that it won't happen. The process of homologous recombination is very inefficient. There's another problem, too—the cell might end up repairing the double-strand break through NHEJ instead of homologous recombination. Instead of the precise deletion or insertion that's desired, NHEJ repair might result in a semi-random mutation.

The upshot is that in the case of the *CCR5* Δ32 deletion, there's no way to ensure that CRISPR-Cas9 will make that exact deletion. And that's a problem if it's important to place that precise deletion into the embryo. A purist would say that it's absolutely necessary to do so; the argument would be as follows. The only mutation that's prevalent in the general population is Δ32. Because one percent of Europeans have two copies of that exact mutation, and they're as healthy as the other ninety-nine percent, we can be sure that putting that mutation into humans will be reasonably safe. We also have strong evidence from studying those one percent of Europeans that two copies of Δ32 will protect against most HIV strains. But we can't say the same about any other mutation—whether it's a thirty-one-base pair deletion, a thirty-three-base pair deletion, a one-base pair deletion, a one-base pair insertion, or anything else. None of them naturally occur in enough living humans that we can be sure that they are both protective against HIV and safe. It's Δ32 or bust.

A pragmatist would push back against this argument and say that as long as we can gather sufficient evidence that mutations other than Δ32 will be protective and safe, it would be reasonable to consider doing the gene editing. (There might be any number of other very good reasons not to do the editing, but the exact nature of the mutations wouldn't be the sticking point.)

Although none of it was discussed in JK's manuscript, there's quite a lot of evidence that many *CCR5* mutations other than Δ32 are protective against HIV. When Dr. Nathaniel Landau and other researchers first published the discovery of the *CCR5* Δ32 mutation in 1996, the company Sangamo BioSciences (now Sangamo Therapeutics) took notice. Sangamo had been founded just the previous year with the goal of using zinc finger technology for therapeutic purposes. *CCR5* was an attractive target. Landau's data suggested that the main effect of the Δ32 mutation was to remove working CCR5 protein from the cell surface where, along with the

CD4 protein, it could otherwise provide a gate through which the HIV virus could enter the cell.

The Sangamo researchers reasoned that any frameshift mutation early in the gene would sufficiently mess up the protein that it would no longer be on the cell surface and be exploited by HIV. If they could get frameshift mutations into both copies of the CCR5 gene in a T cell, then that cell would become resistant to HIV. So Sangamo designed ZFNs that would target the site of the fifty-fifth amino acid of the CCR5 protein. (The Δ32 mutation occurs at the site of the 184th amino acid of CCR5.)

Sangamo then teamed up with Dr. Carl June, an immunologist and oncologist at the University of Pennsylvania. They delivered the ZFNs into human CD4-bearing T cells and then exposed one batch of the cells, but not another batch, to HIV. Only a small percent of the non-HIV-exposed cells had editing of the CCR5 gene. In contrast, the vast majority of the HIV-exposed cells had editing of the gene. This meant that the virus had killed most of the unedited cells, whereas the edited cells were resistant and survived. When the researchers sequenced the CCR5 target site in the genomes of the HIV-exposed cells, they found a huge variety of deletions and insertions, ranging in size from one to forty-three base pairs.

Many of the edits resulted in frameshift mutations, as expected. But quite a few were deletions or insertions with sizes that were multiples of three (three, nine, eighteen, and so on). These mutations would result in removal or insertion of amino acids without otherwise disturbing the rest of the amino acids in the protein. It didn't matter—that was enough to inactivate the protein and confer HIV resistance. Finally, the researchers transplanted gene-edited and unedited T cells into mice and exposed the mice to HIV. After fifty days, the mice that received the edited cells had more T cells and lower amounts of virus in the blood than the mice with the unedited cells. This was proof in living animals that gene editing of CCR5 to produce mutations other than Δ32 offered protection against HIV. The work was published in the journal *Nature Biotechnology* in 2008.

The success of this study inspired Sangamo, June, and Dr. Pablo Tebas at the University of Pennsylvania to carry out a clinical trial with HIV patients. They first needed to provide evidence to the U.S. Food and Drug Administration that the non-Δ32 mutations were protective against HIV. The results from the 2008 study were persuasive enough to allow the trial to go forward. The researchers recruited HIV-positive patients and, for each patient, isolated CD4-bearing T cells from the blood. They used the same ZFNs from the 2008 study to target *CCR5* in the T cells in the dish and then put those cells back into the patient. There were signs that the strategy worked. Edited cells persisted in the bloodstream for a significantly longer time than unedited cells, suggesting they were protected from the virus already in the patient's bodies. In one patient, the virus disappeared from the bloodstream for the entirety of the study. None of the patients were cured—this was expected since healthy T cells have a natural lifespan of months, so the edited cells would not stick around forever even if they were resistant to HIV. Yet the results were encouraging. A preliminary report of the clinical trial was published in the *New England Journal of Medicine* in 2014.

To achieve something closer to a cure, Sangamo had begun working with Dr. Paula Cannon at the University of Southern California in Los Angeles to use the ZFNs to target *CCR5* in bone marrow stem cells rather than T cells. (Bone marrow stem cells are different from embryonic stem cells in that they're not pluripotent. They can only turn into the various blood cells—platelets, red blood cells, and white blood cells, which include T cells—not all of the different cell types throughout the body.) The thinking: if a patient's stem cells are taken out of the body, edited with the ZFNs, and then placed back into the body, the edited stem cells will remain in the bone marrow permanently—similar to the Berlin patient after he received bone marrow transplants from a double-Δ32 donor—and continuously pump out HIV-resistant T cells. In a study published in *Nature Biotechnology* in 2010, Cannon and Sangamo reported that the strategy worked well in mice.

Since CRISPR-Cas9 first arrived on the scene in early 2013, many researchers have jumped at the opportunity to use the new gene editor on *CCR5* in T cells, including me and my collaborators. My survey of the scientific literature found that researchers have succeeded in conferring HIV resistance by targeting any of the following sites with CRISPR-Cas9: the 38th amino acid, the 93rd amino acid, the 105th amino acid, the 153rd amino acid, the 184th amino acid, the 209th amino acid, and the 334th amino acid. No doubt I'm missing some sites from this list. Even so, all of these results suggest that using NHEJ repair to introduce semi-random frameshift mutations at any of a variety of sites in *CCR5* will have a protective effect. There doesn't seem to be anything special about the Δ32 mutation.

Although JK chose not to try to precisely reproduce the *CCR5* Δ32 mutation in the embryos, his strategy of using NHEJ repair to introduce semi-random mutations at the site of the Δ32 mutation did have support from the scientific literature. I couldn't categorically fault him on that score.

The manuscript stated that JK's team had "carefully evaluated the safety and efficiency of *CCR5* gene editing ... in mouse, monkey, donated nonviable human embryos and human embryonic stem cells." It concluded that there was no obvious safety issue. But none of those data were presented in this manuscript: "The preclinical study is published separately in a companion paper." It seemed that JK was writing a second manuscript, one that wasn't accessible to me. But I already had a good idea what was in it.

In July 2007, JK had uploaded to YouTube a video of a presentation he'd given at a scientific conference at Cold Spring Harbor Laboratory on Long Island, New York. The title of his presentation: "Evaluating the safety of germline genome editing in human, monkey, and mouse embryos." I watched the video after finding it on YouTube. It was not reassuring. It showed that there was a huge problem with mosaicism—by JK's own admission, the majority of the embryos he was trying to edit had clear signs of it. He'd suggested a couple of strategies that might reduce the rate of mosaicism, but it wasn't clear that he'd actually done anything to implement them in his clinical trial.

Back to the manuscript. Finally, there was some nuts-and-bolts information about the gene-edited babies. JK's team had collected twelve egg cells from the prospective mother, and they had washed sperm cells from the father to make sure they were clean of HIV virus. They had injected the sperm into the eggs to fertilize them to make zygotes and then had injected CRISPR-Cas9 into the zygotes. They had maintained the zygotes in a dish to allow them to grow over the next five to six days into blastocysts; only four embryos had made it that far. At that point, each embryo would have had two to three hundred cells. The team then had taken three to five cells from each embryo and extracted genomic DNA from those cells. At that point, they had performed two types of sequencing: Sanger sequencing of the CRISPR-Cas9 target site in *CCR5*, and next-generation sequencing of the entire genome. This would have revealed whether the desired editing had occurred and also provided an opportunity to search the genome for off-target mutations.

The manuscript then stated that two of the four blastocysts were successfully edited, and the other two were not. One embryo was edited on both copies of the *CCR5* gene, with each edit being a frameshift mutation: a one-base pair insertion and a four-base pair deletion (neither is a multiple of three). The other embryo was edited on only one copy of the *CCR5* gene, with a fifteen-base pair deletion; the other copy was normal. The fifteen-base pair deletion wasn't a frameshift mutation, since it was a multiple of three. Instead, it would result in the removal of five amino acids from the middle of the protein. The manuscript claimed: "Based on the CCR5 protein structure, this [fifteen-base pair] deletion should effectively disable the CCR5 receptor for HIV." It didn't provide any evidence for this statement. There was an additional claim, that "the [single] *CCR5* edit is expected to confer partial resistance to HIV," similar to having a single copy of the Δ32 mutation.

After learning all this information, I mentally summed things up. The first embryo had two frameshift mutations at the site of the Δ32 mutation. Based on the scientific literature, both mutations were almost certain to inactivate the CCR5 protein and, together, prevent most strains of HIV from infecting T cells.

The second embryo had one working copy of *CCR5* and one 15-base pair deletion. This would result in T cells having some normal protein and some protein missing five amino acids. Would the incomplete protein still work properly? It was hard to know for sure. Think back to the example from Chapter 2: "The quick brown fox jumps over the lazy dog." If you remove the five letters in the word "brown": "The quick fox jumps over the lazy dog." The sentence has more or less the same meaning. But if you remove the five letters in the word "jumps:" "The quick brown fox over the lazy dog." The sentence no longer works. Either scenario might apply to the CCR5 protein missing five amino acids.

But then I realized that it really didn't matter. The manuscript's claim that the single 15-base pair deletion should confer partial resistance to HIV wasn't supported by the scientific literature. People with a single copy of the Δ32 mutation don't actually seem to be resistant, even partly resistant, to an initial infection by the HIV virus. Rather, the time of progression from the initial infection to full-blown AIDS seems to be slower. This might seem like a distinction without a difference, but it's not, for a very important reason—we now have very effective antiviral medications that can stave off AIDS indefinitely. HIV infection is no longer a death sentence. So the benefit of a single copy of the Δ32 mutation isn't as relevant now as it would have been in the 1980s and 1990s. For the second embryo, whether the fifteen-base pair deletion inactivates the protein or not wasn't that important, because there was already one normal copy of the *CCR5* gene. Either way, a child born from that embryo wouldn't be protected against HIV infection and, if she were unfortunate enough to become infected in her lifetime, would benefit from antiviral medications just as anybody else would.

Which, in my mind, immediately raised the question: if the objective of this clinical trial was to "provide newborns with lifelong protection against HIV infection," what would be the point of using the second embryo to establish a pregnancy? There was no way that newborn was going to have lifelong protection against HIV infection, with only partial editing.

Disturbed, I kept reading. The next paragraph was about off-target effects—mutations occurring at sites other than the *CCR5* gene. The manuscript stated that the first embryo didn't show any such mutations. Then, a shocker: the second embryo showed an off-target one-base pair insertion in a region on chromosome 1 (*CCR5* is located on chromosome 3). This directly contradicted the statement in the abstract: "No off-targets, large deletions or pathogenic cancer gene mutations was observed." Yet the manuscript was now admitting there was at least one off-target mutation. But it went on to say that the mutation was far away from any known gene, and "so we concluded that this intergenic off-target genomic insertion might not impact any biological function." This was a clear safety issue—JK didn't know for sure that this mutation wasn't a problem. But he dismissed it out of hand.

The next paragraph raised ethical red flags rather than scientific ones: "After informing the volunteer couples of all the genetic information gleaned from the embryos, including the availability of a viable unedited embryo without detected off-target effects and the potential risk that off-target effects in all of the embryos may not have been detected, the parents chose to have both edited embryos implanted." I had trouble wrapping my head around the notion that any parents would be pleased to be told that their embryo, and therefore their future child, had a known unwanted mutation and might have additional undetected mutations. Had the parents really understood what was going on when presented with this choice?

The manuscript then described the pregnancy. JK's team had taken blood samples from the mother at weeks twelve, nineteen, and twenty-four of the pregnancy. They had probed all of the DNA isolated from the blood samples, looking for traces of DNA that didn't match up with the mother's DNA. Any mismatched DNA, they assumed, came from the pregnancy. JK stated there was evidence of three different *CCR5* edits—the one-base pair insertion and four-base pair deletion matching the first embryo, and the fifteen-base pair deletion matching the second embryo. Would JK's team have done anything differently if they had found evidence of unwanted edits? Would they have advised the parents to abort the fetuses?

Finally, the babies had been born: "normal, healthy twin girls, named Lulu and Nana, in November 2018 in China." (I assumed these were pseudonyms to protect the identities of the babies and their parents.) The manuscript noted that at the time of birth, the placenta, umbilical cord, and umbilical cord blood had been collected for each twin. Nana had apparently come from the first embryo, and Lulu from the second embryo: "We confirmed Nana's *CCR5* gene was edited successfully with frameshift mutations on both [copies] and Lulu's [had the] 15 bp deletion." There was a statement that "no off-target or large deletion was detected in either twin by whole genome deep sequencing." But the sequencing was done only with the placenta and umbilical cord samples. Oddly, there was no mention of sequencing done from the twins' bodies—blood, saliva, or any other tissue. Did JK's team not have access to the actual babies themselves?

The next paragraph described a plan to "further confirm the resistance of each twin to HIV." JK's team wouldn't be doing this by actually administering the virus to the twins and seeing whether they became infected, as that would be monstrously unethical. Instead, they'd be taking T cells from the twins' blood and seeing if HIV could infect the cells outside of the body. This would be a safe way of indirectly assessing the twins' vulnerability to HIV. The manuscript also mentioned a plan to monitor for long-term consequences of the gene editing for at least the next eighteen years, with the hope that the grown-up twins would then consent to continued monitoring throughout their adulthood. This highlighted yet another ethical concern for me, that the twins didn't have any say in whether they should have been edited as embryos. How much consideration had JK given to how the twins might come to feel about the fact that they had been edited?

I reached the end of the main text of the manuscript. "More broadly, however, *CCR5* gene editing provides a conservative first model case for assessing therapeutic gene editing in embryos ..." But there was no justification why editing *CCR5* for a preventable and treatable disease like HIV was a good model case, as opposed to fixing some grievous genetic disorder where a child would otherwise inevitably suffer. "In the future, we hope gene editing in embryos will continue to prove safe and effective at other genomic loci and bring new hope for the prevention and treatment of many genetic diseases." This sentence struck an odd note, since HIV wasn't a genetic disease. The last sentence: "However, for ethical and moral reasons, we believe firmly that the technology should not be used for attempted non-medical genetic modification, such as athletic performance, skin color, sex selection, or intelligence." Was JK trying to better justify his questionable choice of *CCR5* and HIV resistance by pointing out that he could have chosen to do something even more questionable?

Tucked away at the end of the manuscript was a short, separate Methods section. There were some notable non-scientific tidbits here. A statement about ethics: "The study was approved in March 2017 by the Medical Ethics Committee of the Shenzhen Harmonicare Women's and Children's Hospital." Clearly JK had been planning his clinical trial for a long time. "We were told that the committee held a comprehensive discussion of risks and benefits before reaching the approval conclusion." This made it sound like none of JK's team members were in the room when the ethics committee discussed the clinical trial. Did the ethics committee have enough knowledge about gene editing to be able to meaningfully discuss the risks and benefits? It seemed unlikely. "During the study, the director of the ethics committee was constantly updated about the state of the clinical trial."

There was then some discussion of the informed consent process, which is supposed to convey the potential benefits and the potential harms from involvement in a clinical trial before the volunteers agree to participate. "HIV-positive participants in the study were recruited by the BaiHuaLin China People Living With HIV/AIDS Alliance." That explained Hua Bai's authorship on the paper. "[The parents] were then engaged in the multi-week consenting process, which involved discussions with several scientific and clinical consultants who highlighted the risk of this first-in-human embryo use of gene editing." With respect to the potential harms: "Particularly, the risks of potential off-target, side effects of IVF [in vitro fertilization], and unknown biological side effects of genetic editing were emphasized." There was no mention in the manuscript of what potential benefits were communicated to the parents.

My conclusions after an initial read of the main text of JK's manuscript were: Nana is probably resistant to HIV; Lulu is definitely not resistant; lots of unanswered questions and concerns about the science and the ethics. But for whatever reason, JK had chosen to put the most important data—several key pictures—in a separate file, a supplementary document, which I'd deferred reading until after I'd skimmed through the main document. I now went through the pictures carefully, one by one. And my world turned upside down.

The first picture had Sanger sequencing chromatograms showing the *CCR5* target site in genomic DNA taken from three to five cells of each of the four embryos (out of the two to three hundred cells present at the blastocyst stage). Embryo 1 was labeled Lulu, embryo 2 was Nana, and embryos 3 and 4 were unlabeled. I looked at the chromatogram for embryo 1.

Wait, what?

The chromatogram was a mess. I instantly saw that there were three versions of the *CCR5* sequence. Lulu was only supposed to have two, the normal version and the version with a fifteen-base pair deletion.

Omigod, omigod, omigod ... the embryo was mosaic! I let out a guttural scream. Fortunately, the door to my office was closed, but who knows what my neighbors heard and thought. *It couldn't be. Could it? Did JK actually use this embryo for pregnancy?*

I looked down to the chromatogram for embryo 2. Nana, who was supposed to have two versions of the *CCR5* gene, one with a one-base pair insertion, the other with a four-base pair deletion.

The second chromatogram showed three versions of the *CCR5* gene. *Also mosaic!* Another involuntary scream.

Having looked at thousands of chromatograms from gene-edited cells, I knew exactly what I was looking at. But I couldn't quite believe it. Maybe I was just confused about what it was these chromatograms represented. Maybe they were mislabeled. Maybe they were from some different experiment. I looked over at the chromatograms for embryos 3 and 4, which JK had claimed to be unedited. They were pristine. Exactly what you'd expect to see if there was no editing. If both copies of the gene were normal, they would be indistinguishable from each other on a chromatogram, and it would look like there was only one version of the gene: a set of nice, clean, single peaks, as shown in Figure 4.

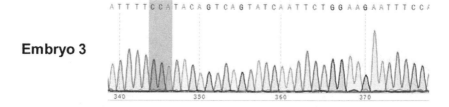

Figure 4

Imagine a scenario where an embryo has one normal copy of *CCR5* and a copy with a one-base pair deletion, and that embryo is not mosaic (all of the cells in the embryo have the same normal copy and deletion copy).

PCR of the site of the mutation would result in roughly equal amplification from the normal copy on one chromosome 3 and from the deletion copy on the other chromosome 3. The final sample would therefore be a roughly equal mix of the two following sequences (underlines indicate differences):

...ATTTTCCATAC<u>A</u>GTCAGTATCAATTCTGGAAGAATTTCC...
...ATTTTCCATAC<u>G</u>TCAGTATCAATTCTGGAAGAATTTCCA...

These sequences march in lockstep until the site of the deletion is reached (the twelfth position in the sequences shown above). After that, the two sequences are no longer in sync.

A chromatogram would show something similar. For the first eleven positions of the sequences shown above—ATTTTCCATAC—there will be single peaks. With the twelfth position—A in the normal sequence, G in the deletion sequence—there will be overlapping peaks of roughly equal height, one for A and one for G. Same for the thirteenth position—G and T. Same for the fourteenth position—T and C. And so forth. Occasionally, there will be a position where the two sequences match by chance; for example, the twenty-second position, where both sequences have A. At that position in the chromatogram there would be a single peak for A. But for the most part, there will be lots of overlapping peaks visible in the chromatogram after the site of the deletion.

Now imagine a scenario where an embryo is mosaic. Half of the cells have one normal copy of *CCR5* and a copy with a one-base pair deletion. The other half of the cells have one normal copy and a copy with a two-base pair deletion. Let's say genomic DNA is made from the entire embryo. PCR of the site of the mutations would result in proportional amplification of the three versions of the gene: two parts normal, one part one-base pair deletion, one part two-base pair deletion. The final sample would therefore be a two-to-one-to-one mix of the following three sequences (underlines indicate differences):

...ATTTTCCATAC<u>A</u>GTCAGTATCAATTCTGGAAGAATTTCC...
...ATTTTCCATAC<u>G</u>TCAGTATCAATTCTGGAAGAATTTCCA...
...ATTTTCCATAC<u>T</u>CAGTATCAATTCTGGAAGAATTTCCAG...

Again, these sequences march in lockstep until the site of the deletion is reached (the twelfth position). After that, the three sequences are no longer in register. On the chromatogram, for the first eleven positions of the sequences shown above, there will be single peaks. With the twelfth position—A in the normal sequence, G in the one-base pair deletion sequence, T in the two-base pair deletion sequence—there will be overlapping peaks, one for A, one for G, and one for T. But we wouldn't expect them to be the same height. The base in the normal sequence—A—would be the dominant peak because it represents about half of the mix. The other bases—G and T—would be smaller peaks because they each represent about a quarter of the mix. These patterns would be apparent at many of the subsequent positions in the chromatogram.

In the chromatogram for embryo 1, there are positions where there clearly are three overlapping peaks, shown in Figure 5 with arrows.

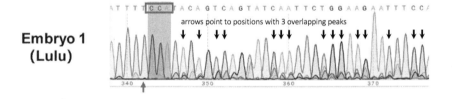

FIGURE 5

There's one dominant set of peaks, which correspond to the normal *CCR5* gene sequence, and two minor sets of peaks. It appears there is a lot more of the normal version of the gene, and less of the other two versions. By playing a kind of sequencing sudoku, it's sometimes possible to parse out the exact identity of multiple sequences on a chromatogram. If the normal sequence is known to be present, subtract out the corresponding peaks and other sequences can be deciphered from the peaks that are left behind. Here it appears that one of the minor sequences has a fifteen-base pair deletion, exactly as claimed by JK. The third sequence is difficult to ascertain, but it appears to have a large insertion.

The best way to explain this chromatogram: out of the three to five cells sampled from the blastocyst and analyzed by sequencing, one cell had one normal *CCR5* copy and one fifteen-base pair deletion copy, one cell had one normal copy and a different edited (insertion?) copy, and the other cell(s) had two normal copies. This is enough to establish the embryo as mosaic.

The chromatogram for embryo 2 also has positions where there are three overlapping peaks, shown in Figure 6 with arrows.

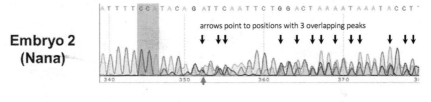

FIGURE 6

Embryo 2 is more complicated than embryo 1. Playing the sequencing sudoku game again, there appear to be three different edited versions (and no normal version): one with a one-base pair insertion and one with a four-base pair deletion (as claimed by JK), and a third one with a large unspecified insertion. No one version is clearly dominant. The best we can conclude is that the three to five cells sampled from the blastocyst were a mix of differently edited cells. This embryo was unambiguously mosaic, too.

By now I was very upset and confused—*what's going on here? both Lulu's and Nana's embryos were mosaic?*—and my mind was reeling from the implications. But I went on to the other pictures. The second picture provided data on the next-generation sequencing performed on the three to five cells sampled from Lulu's and Nana's blastocysts. The intent had been to scan the entire genome for off-target effects. But this picture made it clear that the sequencing hadn't worked so well. For each embryo, it only covered about half of the genome at a level of sufficiently high quality to reliably detect unintended mutations. Any off-target effects in the remainder of the genome could have been missed.

The third picture showed another chromatogram, this one confirming the single off-target effect that JK's team had detected with the next-generation sequencing. This was the mutation in Lulu's embryo that JK had dismissed as being too far away from any gene to be of any concern. He had described it as a one-base pair insertion mutation on chromosome 1, so I assumed it meant that there was one copy of the mutated sequence, with one normal copy of that sequence on the other chromosome 1. I was expecting the chromatogram to show overlapping peaks of roughly equal height starting from the position of the one-base pair insertion.

The chromatogram shows the overlapping peaks, all right, but it also provides yet more evidence of mosaicism in Lulu's embryo, shown in Figure 7.

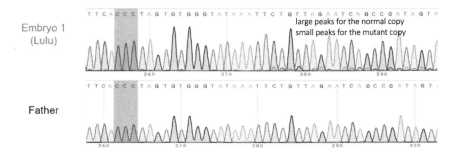

FIGURE 7

There is clearly a mutated version of the gene present (compare Lulu's chromatogram to the totally normal chromatogram from the father), but there appears to be a lot more of the normal version and a lot less of the mutant version. The most plausible scenario: out of the three to five cells sampled from the blastocyst and analyzed by sequencing, one cell had one normal copy of the sequence and one 1-base pair insertion copy, and the other cells had two normal copies. My conclusion: Lulu's embryo was not only mosaic at the intended *CCR5* target site, but was also mosaic for an unintended mutation elsewhere in the genome. This was starting to look like a real hack job. At the same time, it wasn't really out of line with what one might expect to happen with CRISPR-Cas9 gene editing, messy as it tends to be.

The fourth picture was the coup de grâce. It included chromatograms for the *CCR5* target site from post-birth samples of umbilical cord blood, umbilical cord, and placenta for each twin. Nana's chromatograms seem straightforward. Each of them shows just two versions of *CCR5*, with overlapping peaks of roughly similar height. The two versions have the reported one-base pair insertion and four-base pair deletion, respectively. No normal version is present.

Lulu's chromatograms are a different story.

The cord blood and umbilical cord samples show two versions of *CCR5*, with overlapping peaks of roughly similar height. With sequencing sudoku, it appears to be what JK reported: a normal version and a fifteen-base pair deletion version. Something quite different is going on in the placenta, though. There are clearly positions with three overlapping peaks, shown in Figure 8 with arrows. Once again, mosaicism rears its ugly head. Close inspection shows that the normal copy and fifteen-base pair deletion copy are present, yet there is another version that is hard to interpret, but appears to have a large insertion.

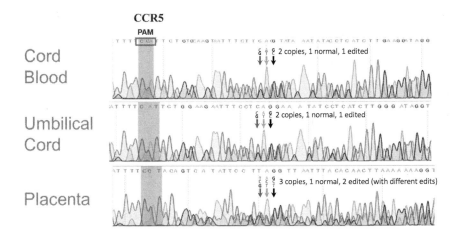

Figure 8

If Lulu's embryo and placenta were both mosaic—the evidence seemed incontrovertible, with three different pictures pointing to the same conclusion—what was the likelihood that Lulu was mosaic in her body? Much higher than zero, I was certain. The same was true for Nana, since her embryo was clearly mosaic as well. But the only way to know for sure would be to take samples from all throughout the babies' bodies. That's the devilish thing about mosaicism. By its nature, it could be affecting some parts of the body but not others. To rule it out would require a battery of invasive procedures on the twins. I couldn't imagine the parents or, once they're old enough, the twins themselves consenting to that.

By the time I finished going through the pictures, I was near tears from a mix of fury and anguish. I was certain now that the twins were real flesh-and-blood human beings. There was no way JK had faked this. If this were a hoax, why would he have included pictures showing that the embryos and placenta were mosaic? He would have used perfect-looking data, which is easy enough to fabricate. In fact, it would be much harder to fabricate chromatograms that showed mosaicism. Not impossible, but it would be truly bizarre to go through that much trouble to undermine your own data if the goal was to convince everybody you'd achieved a world first.

Both embryos were flawed. That thought reverberated in my head, over and over, as adrenaline surged through my body. Why on earth had JK proceeded with two flawed embryos? There were just two alternatives. The first was incompetence. Neither JK nor anybody on his team knew how to interpret chromatograms. They hadn't realized the implications of their own data. They had thought everything was fine, despite being well aware of the propensity of CRISPR-Cas9 to cause mosaicism, and proceeded with the pregnancy. The second was wanton disregard. JK had understood the chromatograms, but he had been so keen on being the first to make gene-edited babies that it simply hadn't mattered to him that the embryos were flawed. He had gone forward with the pregnancy, willing to take the chance that any live-born children might suffer serious consequences. If so, it was a sign of monstrous inhumanity.

I wasn't sure which explanation was worse. Not that it really mattered. Both were truly awful. The enormity of the situation hit me hard. I wanted to scream; I wanted to cry. The knowledge that somebody had gone ahead and made the first gene-edited babies—for better or for worse, a historic event for humankind—would have been distressing enough, even if it had been done perfectly. The fact that it had been done with flawed embryos, in such a careless fashion, made it a hundred times worse.

9

THE SUMMIT

I couldn't believe it. I went over the chromatograms again and again to be sure I hadn't missed something. But the conclusion was inescapable. The first attempt to hack the code of life and, ostensibly, improve the health of human babies had in fact been a hack job.

It was time to share the bad news with Marilynn Marchione of the Associated Press. In a long email, I explained my conclusions about the gene-edited twins and the reasons supporting those conclusions. There were many unanswered questions, but perhaps the most important one was what the mosaicism meant for the health of the twins. My horror at the fact that JK had used mosaic embryos to establish a pregnancy notwithstanding, was it really going to be a problem for Lulu and Nana?

When JK's team took three to five cells from a blastocyst of two to three hundred cells and subjected those few cells to intensive analysis, they were assuming that whatever was present in those few cells (*CCR5* mutations) was also present in all the rest of the cells of the embryo. Just as importantly, they were assuming that whatever was absent in those few cells (off-target mutations) was also absent in all of the other cells. The problem with mosaicism is that it undermines those assumptions. The few sampled cells could look perfect, but there could be problems in the rest of the blastocyst. And it's the rest of the blastocyst—not the sampled cells—that ultimately becomes a live-born child.

JK knew, or should have known, that even just the three to five cells taken from each embryo showed signs of mosaicism. Think about what that means. If there were differences among just those few cells, how many differences might have been present across the remaining two to three hundred cells in the blastocyst? They might have been a rampant patchwork of different mutations. And JK had no way of knowing if that was the case or not. He had rolled the dice by taking the two embryos through pregnancy.

As we saw in Chapter 7, having just a few percent of cells in the heart carrying a harmful mutation—the smallest taint in the body—was enough to cause a life-threatening condition for a newborn child and require a heart transplant six months later. To be fair, there was no indication that the twins weren't healthy. But I could envision two long-term issues that might have profound implications for their future health.

First, the premise of the gene editing had been to confer resistance to HIV infection. Lulu never had a chance at that, since at best only one of her copies of the CCR5 gene has a mutation. Regardless of the effect of the mutation, having one normal copy of the gene ensures that Lulu is vulnerable to the virus. Nana, with frameshift mutations in both copies of the CCR5 gene that were almost certain to prevent any working protein from being made, does have a chance at resistance to most HIV strains. But that assumes that every cell in her body has the two frameshift mutations. What if some proportion of her cells, even a small proportion, have only one frameshift mutation or even no frameshift mutation due to mosaicism? If Nana were to be exposed to HIV at some point in her life, those cells might be enough to allow HIV to gain a foothold in her body. She might be infected after all, and perhaps even be able to pass the virus on to other people. There's even a perverse scenario where upon learning about her gene-edited condition and believing she's resistant to HIV, Nana might feel emboldened to engage in risky behaviors that expose her to the virus, to which her mosaic body might then succumb.

Second, there's the possibility of off-target effects of the gene editing. It was already clear from JK's presentation that Lulu's embryo had at least one unanticipated mutation, on a different chromosome than the *CCR5* gene. Indeed, that one mutation appeared to be mosaic, probably present in just one of the three to five cells sampled from Lulu's blastocyst. What other unanticipated mutations had been hidden away in Lulu's and Nana's blastocysts? Did any such mutation end up in either of the twins' bodies? The mutation wouldn't need to be in all of the child's cells to cause a problem. We already know it can happen with heart disease. It certainly can happen with other diseases, with cancer being the most serious concern.

Cancer typically starts with one cell. The cell picks up a harmful mutation, then one of its descendant cells picks up a second harmful mutation, then one of that cell's descendant cells picks up a third harmful mutation, and so on until the mutations together have caused the cell to grow wildly out of control into a tumor and to spread across the body. It typically takes years or decades to accumulate the necessary number of mutations to have full-blown cancer cells. An off-target effect might supply some of the cells in the child's body—even if only a few cells hidden away deep in the body, impossible to detect—with the first needed mutation and substantially accelerate the timeline to cancer.

It would be particularly tragic if Lulu were to develop a disease like cancer as a result of the gene editing performed on her embryo, when she was never in a position to benefit from the HIV resistance that was the purported goal of the editing.

I was struck by an even more ominous possibility. What if a harmful mutation had ended up in some of the cells of one of the twins' bodies, including some of her egg cells? In the twin herself, the mutation might not be present in enough of her cells to cause disease. Her mosaicism might protect her. But each egg cell has the potential to become a whole human being. If the egg cell carried the mutation, so too would a zygote arising from that egg cell, and so too would the embryo arising from that zygote, and so too would the child born from the embryo. And that child would not be mosaic—every single one of her cells would have the harmful mutation. So even though the twin might be fortunate enough to escape disease and have no inkling that the mutation is lurking in her body, her own child could suffer from it. The consequences of mosaicism might extend to future generations.

It is possible—indeed, it is to be fervently prayed—that Lulu and Nana and their children will suffer none of the ill consequences of mosaicism. But even if that fortunate outcome should come to pass, the ends would not justify the means. The potential risks are real. And they're also devilishly difficult to define, precisely because the medical community has never faced this situation before: mosaicism resulting from a deliberate manmade intervention. JK should have been far more mindful of the unknown dangers of mosaicism, and they should have deterred him from establishing a pregnancy.

Besides the issue of mosaicism, I had three major concerns. They all centered on the choice of *CCR5* as the target gene. It initially baffled me that JK's team proceeded to pregnancy with Lulu's embryo. There are many people in the general population who have one copy of the *CCR5* Δ 32 mutation—indeed, about ten percent of Europeans. The most definitive research concerning these people has found no protection from an initial HIV infection. Older data from the 1990s, when antiviral therapies were still new, suggested that after the initial infection an HIV carrier might progress more slowly to AIDS. But today's antiviral therapies halt the progression to AIDS, irrespective of whether a Δ32 mutation is present or not.

Furthermore, the one *CCR5* mutation that Lulu does carry (putting aside the possibility of mosaicism) causes a five-amino-acid deletion of questionable effect on the CCR5 protein. It's quite possible that Lulu is no different from the average individual with two normal copies of *CCR5*. There really was no medical justification for JK's team to offer Lulu's embryo to the parents, when there was no chance of HIV resistance and very much a chance of unintended harms from the experimental gene-editing procedure. Later on, I realized that it would only make sense to proceed with Lulu's embryo if the goal was to maximize the chance of the world's first gene-edited baby being born, even if the editing offered no benefit whatsoever. Pregnancies with in vitro fertilization are chancy, with most implanted embryos not making it to birth. JK might have been thinking that if only Lulu and not Nana was born, he would still earn bragging rights for a historic scientific accomplishment.

Nana was a different story. Given that she has two inactivating frameshift mutations in *CCR5* (again putting aside the possibility of mosaicism), I was fairly certain she'd enjoy as much resistance to HIV infection as the one percent of Europeans who have two Δ32 mutations. But would it actually benefit her? She had no exposure to the virus while in the womb or during childbirth, as her mother was HIV-negative. She has minimal chance of being exposed to the virus during childhood. Simply having an HIV-positive father wouldn't promote transmission of the virus through casual contact, and he's been on antiviral therapy and free of virus in his bloodstream in any case.

If Nana hadn't been edited as an embryo, her risk of contracting the virus during her lifetime would have been no different than any of her peers—exceedingly small. The prevalence of HIV infection in China is less than one tenth of one percent. The primary routes are sexual transmission, drug use, and blood transfusions, with the last one largely eliminated due to nationwide screening of the blood supply. Even if she somehow were to become infected with HIV, she would be able to receive antiviral therapy like her father. That's not even considering new advances in HIV research that might emerge over the next few decades, such as curative therapy for HIV or an HIV vaccine. The upshot is that Nana's chance of suffering from

AIDS in her lifetime is close to zero. Her gene editing didn't do much to reduce an already negligible risk.

On the other hand, Nana might actually suffer serious harm from having two *CCR5* mutations. We have *CCR5* for a reason. It turns out to be important in fighting off viral infections besides HIV. The best established is West Nile virus, which is transmitted by mosquitoes. People who have two Δ32 mutations suffer a more serious illness if they have the viral infection, though it's not clear whether they're more prone to being infected in the first place. (Most patients infected with West Nile virus have no symptoms and don't know they're infected.) The same is true of tick-borne encephalitis virus—two Δ32 mutations increase the risk of severe brain infection with viral infection. Both West Nile virus and tick-borne encephalitis virus infections are rare in urban areas of China, rarer than HIV. Moreover, vaccines against tick-borne encephalitis virus have been in use in China for decades. So one could reasonably question whether Nana's increased risk with these viruses is meaningful.

What cannot be questioned as easily is the risk from influenza viruses, which cause garden-variety flu. Multiple studies have shown that having two Δ32 mutations greatly increases the risk of dying from flu. It's also well established that mice lacking the CCR5 protein are more vulnerable to death from flu. Flu is very common, with millions of cases of severe flu illness and hundreds of thousands of deaths worldwide each year despite the availability of flu vaccines. The deaths disproportionately occur in very young and old people, but healthy individuals in their twenties can die of flu too. Unlike the other viruses, transmission of flu occurs quite readily with casual contact. Flu is as much a problem in China as it is anywhere else in the world. Indeed, the origins of some flu epidemics have been traced to China.

So the chance of Nana getting flu is substantial, far higher than the risk of HIV infection. And if the editing performed on her embryo makes her more likely to die of flu, as the available evidence suggests, that's a substantial health concern that shouldn't be dismissed. It would be one thing if a person inherited two Δ32 mutations from her parents and dies from flu for that reason—that is bad luck. It would be another thing entirely if a person's embryo was deliberately manipulated and it results in death from flu.

I had already scheduled a video interview with the Associated Press for the following afternoon (the Tuesday before Thanksgiving). I spent the evening and the next morning thinking about what I should say. I was daunted about the interview. I realized that besides JK himself, I'd likely be having the first word on the gene-edited twins in the eyes of the world. There was never any question that I was going to strongly condemn what JK had done. But I didn't want any of my tumultuous emotions seething just beneath the surface to erupt during the interview. Then I'd risk coming across as a bit unhinged and, perhaps, not credible. I needed to be stern but measured in my response. I also needed to make sure that I communicated the complicated issues at play in a clear and concise way, since I assumed clips of the video interview might be broadcast widely. Fortunately, the interview ended up going smoothly.

With all of this going on, any chance of my getting any work done that wasn't related to gene-edited babies was shot. Indeed, I was in a perpetual state of distraction for the rest of the week. When I went to my computer to try to do unrelated tasks, I found myself taking another look at the manuscript and obsessing over whether I'd missed anything. Even when not at work, no matter what I tried to do, my thoughts kept coming back to the twins. I had trouble sleeping. I must have been terrible company during the Thanksgiving holiday that week. My general demeanor must have broadcast my distress, because a number of people asked me what was wrong. But being sworn to confidentiality, I couldn't discuss the twins with anybody. I had to handwave and make excuses.

When I was given JK's manuscript, I had the opportunity to e-mail JK and ask him scientific questions about the work. I was briefly tempted to write to him and demand to know what had possessed him to use flagrantly mosaic embryos for a pregnancy, or if he even understood the implications of his own data. But I decided that I didn't want to engage this man in any way and in some fashion become complicit in his work. There was the possibility that if I pointed out the flawed chromatograms to him, his response might be to replace them with clean-looking ones. The last thing I wanted to do was help him strengthen the presentation of his work when he unveiled it to the world.

The days dragged on without my learning much new. At this point it was just a matter of stewing in secrecy, waiting until JK's presentation at the Second International Summit on Human Genome Editing in Hong Kong in a few days. Then I finally could talk openly. But by the weekend after Thanksgiving, the awful thought had occurred to me: what if JK says nothing at all about Lulu and Nana at the Summit? Maybe he would decide that it would be better to wait until after the Summit. It would give him the chance to do more studies on the twins, write a more comprehensive manuscript, publish the work in a scientific journal, and perhaps be more in control of a publicity rollout.

Then I would be in an impossibly difficult position. How long could I remain silent about the work, knowing with virtual certainty that Lulu and Nana were real human beings and that, in my view, terrible things had been done to them? I was already fit to burst with very strong emotions about the affair. I was staying silent only because I had sworn to do so and because my impression was the news would be out very soon. But I wasn't sure I'd be able to keep quiet much longer. Nor did I think it would be ethical and moral to do so. The burden of knowledge weighed on me in a way I had never experienced before, and I couldn't sleep a wink at night.

I thank my lucky stars that fate and Antonio Regalado intervened when they did.

Regalado, senior editor for biomedicine for *MIT Technology Review*, had been chasing his story for a while. Just the previous month, October 2018, he had taken a trip to China to interview various Chinese scientists who had published studies on human embryo editing. Part of his intent, no doubt, was to nose about for any evidence that someone was taking the work beyond editing of embryos to actual pregnancy. But he hadn't turned up any such evidence.

In any case, Regalado continued to keep close track of what was happening in China after returning from his trip. During the weekend after Thanksgiving, while he was doing research on the Internet, a fortuitous Google search turned up something new—documentation of a post-registered clinical trial by a Dr. He Jiankui titled "Safety and validity evaluation of HIV immune gene CCR5 gene editing in human embryos" on the Chinese Clinical Trial Registry website, dated November 8, 2018. This was the very same web page I had inspected less than a week earlier. From the documents, Regalado could tell that JK had been actively recruiting couples for a trial with human embryo editing. What wasn't immediately clear was whether the clinical trial had actually gotten underway yet.

Then Regalado found the smoking gun. Tucked away in the documentation was the same spreadsheet I had noticed earlier—one full of data about DNA sequences and DNA variants, including the annotations of "Maternal Blood 12 Weeks," "Maternal Blood 19 Weeks," and "Maternal Blood 24 Weeks." From the data in the spreadsheet, Regalado deduced that there were two fetuses at least twenty-four weeks in progress, placing them in the second trimester of pregnancy. While it wasn't enough to conclude that gene-edited babies had been born, it was enough to spur Regalado into action. He unsuccessfully reached out to JK for comment and then wrote a comprehensive piece about the clinical trial, the pregnancy, and JK's backstory. It was published under the title "EXCLUSIVE: Chinese scientists are creating CRISPR babies" on the evening of Sunday, November 25, in the

United States. In Hong Kong, it was the morning of Monday, November 26—the day before the Summit was to begin. JK's thunder had been stolen.

A couple of hours after Regalado's article was published, the Associated Press published Marchione's article reporting on JK's claim of the world's first gene-edited babies. The article did a marvelous job of explaining the details of JK's efforts to produce the babies; the intensive work Marchione and her colleagues at the Associated Press had put into the story showed clearly. I learned some details for the first time. Apparently, Lulu's and Nana's parents weren't the only couple who'd enrolled in JK's clinical trial; six other couples had participated. A total of twenty-two human embryos from the couples were treated with CRISPR-Cas9; sixteen of the embryos had edits in the *CCR5* gene; eleven embryos were used in six attempts to establish a pregnancy before the successful one that resulted in the birth of Lulu and Nana. The scope of JK's clinical trial had been much more extensive than I'd realized.

At first blush, the article might have appeared to be a standard news piece reporting a scientific advancement. It included a series of photos taken by the Associated Press team at JK's laboratory and featuring members of JK's team. Standard shots of scientists doing science: holding instruments, gazing into microscopes, looking intently at computer screens. Though I didn't notice it at the time, several of the photos had captions that mentioned the researchers were working with CRISPR-Cas9 targeting *PCSK9* in human embryos—an oddity given that the twins had been edited in the *CCR5* gene for HIV resistance. The Associated Press produced an accompanying video featuring clips of JK speaking as the lead researcher and giving a lay-friendly explanation of the CRISPR-Cas9 technology and how it edited the embryos resulting in the twins.

Yet in no way did the article serve to cheerlead or promote JK's work. At the beginning of the article, it stated that JK's claim, if true, "would be a profound leap of science and ethics." Immediately after JK's first quote, that "I feel a strong responsibility that it's not just to make a first, but also make it an example," I was quoted with my unequivocal condemnation, that what JK had done was "unconscionable ... an experiment on human beings that is not morally or ethically defensible." A quote by Dr. Eric Topol at the Scripps Research Translational Institute in California followed: "This is far too premature ... We're dealing with the operating instructions of a human being. It's a big deal." Then a somewhat contrarian take by Dr. George Church at Harvard Medical School that with HIV being "a major and growing public health threat ... I think this is justifiable." My statement was by far the strongest denunciation in the article, in no small part fueled by my anger that JK had used flawed embryos for the pregnancy that resulted in the twins. In the accompanying video, the clips of JK justifying the work were interspersed with clips of me roundly criticizing the work.

I might have been the first to publicly criticize the work, but it was just a harbinger of the tsunami to come. The condemnation descended from all quarters, near universal. Much of it came from JK's fellow Chinese scientists, with more than one hundred of them co-signing an open letter calling his clinical trial "crazy" the same day the news broke.

As it happened, I was asleep when Regalado's and Marchione's articles were published in quick succession and the rest of the world started to respond. For the first time in days, the fatigue from sleepless nights had overwhelmed me that Sunday evening. I didn't know what was afoot until about 4 a.m., when I woke up and checked my email on my phone, which was lying on my nightstand—and the inbox had dozens of new messages. Even before I saw any of the subject lines, I knew it could mean only one thing. The news about the gene-edited babies had broken overnight. Sure enough, the messages were almost all inquiries from journalists. The overwhelming emotion I felt at that moment was relief. That huge burden of secret knowledge was lifted from my shoulders. Now I could tell anyone what I knew and exactly how I felt about it.

The action for the next few days was centered at the Second International Summit on Human Genome Editing in Hong Kong. Sharon Begley and Andrew Joseph, journalists at *STAT* (a news site for health, medicine, and scientific discovery), were able to reconstruct the events leading up to JK's scheduled presentation on Wednesday afternoon through onsite interviews and other investigative reporting.

Regalado's article in *MIT Technology Review* dropped like a bombshell on the eve of the Summit. JK requested a meeting with Dr. Jennifer Doudna of the University of California, Berkeley, one of the organizers of the Summit. JK had been invited to present at the Summit with the understanding that he would be presenting his work on gene editing in mouse, monkey, and human embryos. The slide presentation that JK submitted to the organizers several weeks before the Summit made no mention of pregnancy. Now JK and Doudna discussed whether he should talk about Lulu and Nana in his presentation. JK agreed to have dinner with Doudna and a few of the other Summit organizers that night to discuss it further. "His demeanor was an odd combination of hubris and naivete," Doudna told *STAT*. "He was very confident in his work, and totally not understanding what an explosion he had caused."

JK had prepared an elaborate public relations campaign to announce the births of Lulu and Nana. He had even hired an American public relations advisor. When Regalado's and Marchione's articles were published, JK released a series of YouTube videos to explain and promote his team's work. One of the videos mentioned an email address well-wishers could use to send messages to the twins: DearLuluAndNana@gmail.com. In multiple videos, he drew parallels between his work and in vitro fertilization, which had first produced a human baby forty years earlier. While in vitro fertilization had been controversial when it was first used, it is now widely accepted and has helped millions of prospective parents. Indeed, in conversations with others, JK frequently invoked the name of Dr. Robert Edward, who co-developed the in vitro fertilization technique and received the Nobel Prize in Physiology or Medicine in 2010. Perhaps JK was signaling that he hoped his own work would have similar impact and be honored in similar fashion.

The immediate reaction was surely not what JK had expected. No doubt he was taken aback by the fierce, widespread condemnation that rained down on him throughout the course of the day. From many of his fellow researchers there was derision for his choice to make the announcement via YouTube rather than through proper scientific channels—namely a peer-reviewed paper in a scientific journal. Southern University of Science and Technology, JK's home institution in Shenzhen, denied all knowledge of JK's clinical trial and announced an investigation.

The dinner that evening did not go smoothly. Not surprisingly, the Summit organizers grilled JK with questions about both the science and the ethics of his clinical trial. After an hour, he had enough; he stormed out of the restaurant. By that point JK was concerned enough about his safety that he switched hotels that night. It was not clear whether he was going to stay in Hong Kong and give his scheduled talk two days later.

The Summit opened the next morning as planned. It was undoubtedly a surreal experience for the attendees. The whole rationale for the Summit was to engage scientists, clinicians, ethicists, policymakers, and other stakeholders from around the world in a discussion about the proper framework through which to carry out research on human embryo editing and to decide under what conditions it might be appropriate to proceed with pregnancy. In one stroke, JK made a mockery of that rationale, rendered some of the talks instantly obsolete, and did it in such a way that the attendees didn't have enough information about JK's activities to meaningfully react to them. The speakers for the first day and a half of the Summit went on with their planned presentations, making oblique references to the elephant in the room—or, in this case, twin elephants with the names Lulu and Nana.

The planned Wednesday early afternoon session of the Summit, titled "Human Embryo Editing," originally was scheduled as a series of five twelve-minute talks, followed by a half-hour panel discussion with the five speakers. JK had been scheduled as the last of the five speakers. Clearly that format was no longer going to work. The revised session was split into two parts. The first part would feature the first four speakers, followed by a panel discussion. The second part would be what had become the main event of the entire Summit: JK's presentation followed by a moderated question-and-answer session. The Summit presentations were being simultaneously webcast, so the audience wasn't limited to the several hundred people who could fit in the auditorium at the University of Hong Kong. Anyone from anywhere in the world could tune in. It was Tuesday night on the East Coast of the United States, and I planned to stay up late to see what JK had to say for himself. But I was also interested in the general science in the session and watched the four preceding presentations.

The first presentation, by Dr. Kathy Niakan of the Francis Crick Institute in London, described the results of her studies on the gene *POU5F1* in early human embryo development. She had no interest in establishing pregnancies, but her work offered an object lesson on the potential dangers of gene editing. She used the same strategy to inactivate *POU5F1* in human embryos that JK had used to inactivate *CCR5* in Lulu's and Nana's embryos—to point CRISPR-Cas9 at the gene and introduce semi-random frameshift mutations via NHEJ repair. Niakin found that the results were quite unpredictable. Some of the embryos had the expected small insertions and deletions. Others had substantially larger changes. In some cases, there was even loss of a whole portion of a chromosome or, oppositely, duplication of a portion of the chromosome, anchored at the location of the *POU5F1* gene. Such a large-scale deletion or duplication would not affect just one gene, it would involve dozens or even hundreds of genes.

The next three presentations and the subsequent panel discussion touched upon various aspects of human embryo editing. Nothing surprising, just extensions on work that had already been published. No doubt the audience members were restless in anticipation of what was to come next. I certainly was.

Finally, it was time for JK's talk. The moderator of the session, Dr. Robin Lovell-Badge of the Francis Crick Institute, spoke for a few minutes to emphasize the need for decorum and to convey that he would not hesitate to stop the session if there were interruptions. He was concerned there would be strong reactions from the audience that might disrupt the proceedings. He also made it clear that the Summit organizers had no idea JK had established pregnancies with edited human embryos until the news had broken a couple of days earlier. He then asked JK to come to the stage and present his work.

The next thirty seconds were awkward. Neither Lovell-Badge nor anybody else in the auditorium seemed to know where JK was. There was polite, scattered clapping from the audience, undoubtedly out of sheer habit rather than indicating any support of JK's forthcoming presentation. After what seemed an interminable wait, JK showed up at one end of the stage and crossed over to the speaker podium, where Lovell-Badge asked him not to speak for too long and then walked off the stage. Before JK even had a chance to begin, the reporters had burst into action. The clicks of the cameras were deafening to those sitting nearby, and as JK spoke his first halting words, Lovell-Badge raised his voice from off-stage to ask the reporters to cool it with the photographs.

JK started his talk on an odd note: "First, I must apologize that these results leaked unexpectedly, taking away from the community of the full data being presented immediately in a scientific venue and through a peer-review process engaged before this conference." There was no suggestion that the last couple of days, with the barrage of criticisms from commentators around the world, had made him question the appropriateness of his actions in pursuing the first gene-edited babies. I was taken aback that JK seemed remorseful only that his thunder was stolen by Antonio Regalado and that he had not been in full control of his story. JK followed that up by saying that he had submitted a manuscript to a scientific journal (later reported to be the journal *Nature*). Presumably this was the manuscript Marchione had sent me the previous week. I wondered how much of the manuscript's data JK would be including in his presentation, and whether he would show anything that I had not seen before. Would he withhold any of the chromatograms that I had found so incriminating?

JK whirled through a barrage of slides, more than fifty, describing his gene-editing studies in mouse embryos, monkey embryos, human embryos, and embryonic stem cells, and then finally the clinical trial that resulted in Lulu and Nana. He described each slide with only a few sentences and then moved on quickly to the next slide. I already had a good idea what was coming, yet I still had trouble following the presentation. I can only imagine how bewildering it must have been to everyone else watching him speak.

I was astonished when I realized that he was showing exactly the same pictures that were in his manuscript, including the problematic chromatograms. *He really must not realize the chromatograms show severe mosaicism,* I thought. *Otherwise he would be crazy to be showing them to the world.* He had made only one change to one of the pictures. He added labeling to the chromatograms from the Sanger sequencing of the *CCR5* target site in the cells sampled from Lulu's and Nana's embryos. Except that he mixed up his labels—he switched the mutations for the twins, making it seem like Lulu had two mutations and Nana only had one. Unbelievably, he had made a careless error on the slide. This inattention was odd, since he must have realized this was the most important talk of his career. In his shoes, I would have slaved over the details of the slides, making sure everything was exactly right for a talk of this magnitude. (The mislabeling led to all sorts of confusion afterward when other researchers tried to understand JK's data by poring over snapshots of his slides taken by audience members.)

At the end of the talk, there was brief, polite applause. Then Lovell-Badge and Dr. Matthew Porteus of Stanford University, another Summit organizer and the co-moderator for the question-and-answer session, walked up on stage. The three men sat down in chairs, the co-moderators flanking JK, each with a microphone in hand. Lovell-Badge and Porteus gently asked a series of questions about the clinical trial and the informed consent process. Some interesting details came out in JK's responses. He claimed that he had consulted with scientists, clinicians, and ethicists, including several in the United States. Yet he also stated that his university, Southern University of Science and Technology, had no knowledge of the clinical trial. The informed consent documents were reviewed by just four people. JK reported that he personally spent an hour and ten minutes getting informed consent from the volunteer couple. He also confirmed that a professor from the United States had observed the consent process. The couple was recruited for the clinical trial by an HIV/AIDS volunteer group.

The co-moderators then opened the floor for questions from audience members. For about thirty minutes, JK was asked about a variety of scientific and ethical concerns. I was most impressed with the questioners. All were respectful, not accusatory in any way. They asked serious questions that conveyed that they were genuinely trying to understand JK's point of view. Several even thanked JK for being willing to speak to them. By the time the session was finished, I felt an immense pride in my fellow scientists. I had no doubt many of the audience members, including some of the questioners, were seething inside and feeling the same anger I'd been experiencing ever since I'd found out about JK's activities. But they all took the high road and remained civil—no noise, no interruptions, not a single harsh tone.

I was much less impressed with JK. In general, his answers were evasive. Through multiple questions about why he had been so secretive about his work, he responded with the same lines about having consulted with a number of experts, including some in the United States. When asked why he chose *CCR5* and HIV: "I have personally experienced with some people in a AIDS village where thirty percent of village people were infected. They even have to give their children to the relatives and uncles to raise just to prevent potential transmission."

This was not a particularly persuasive rationale for his clinical trial. It was well documented that the reason for such high prevalence in many rural villages in China was not because of unmet medical need or because of rampant transmission of HIV from parents to the children they were raising. Rather, it was because of corrupt exploitation of the desperately poor villagers. They had been paid to donate their blood through blood stations, some legal, most illegal. The blood from many donors had been pooled. Plasma had been extracted from the pooled blood so it could be resold at a profit. And then the remainder of the blood—now all contaminated with HIV from a few of the donors—had been injected back into the donors so they would be able to give blood again more quickly and ring up more profits for the blood stations. The consequences had been catastrophic and easily avoidable.

Perhaps the most remarkable of JK's responses, referring to the parents of the twins: "And also for this specific case, I feel proud, actually. I feel proudest, because [the father] thought that he lost hope for the life. But when the babies were born, with this protection, he sent a message at their birth saying I will work hard, earn money, and take care of his two daughters and his wife ..." I had to wonder whether what had really happened was that the couple were desperate for children, period, rather than being desperate for HIV-resistant children. JK's clinical trial might have been the only way they would have access to in vitro fertilization and become parents. It smacked of potential exploitation.

The biggest bombshell of the evening came when Porteus asked JK point-blank if there were any other pregnancies in progress as part of his clinical trials. After some hesitation, JK admitted there was another early-stage pregnancy. He did not volunteer any more details.

Perhaps the most thoughtful line of questioning came at the end of the session from Dr. Maria Jasin of the Sloan Kettering Institute. She was concerned about how the twins would be viewed by their parents and how they would come to view themselves. Because Nana would be resistant to

HIV infection and Lulu would not, would they be treated differently by their parents and relatives? Would Nana be more desirable as a spouse? Their status as gene-edited children might affect their upbringing. Had JK given any thought to these issues?

JK was taken aback, flummoxed. Clearly he hadn't given much consideration to these issues at all. "I don't know how to answer this question."

10

UNWELCOME CONNECTIONS

On the day after JK's Summit presentation, Dr. Xu Nanping, China's vice minister of science and technology—effectively the Chinese government's official spokesperson on the matter—was quoted by the state broadcaster China Central Television as saying that JK "blatantly violated China's relevant laws and regulations" and "the bottom line of morality and ethics that the academic community adheres to." JK's work had been suspended and was under investigation by the government. "It is shocking and unacceptable," said Xu. "We are resolutely opposed to it."

After his presentation, JK wasn't seen in public for a full month. There were rumors he was under house arrest by Chinese authorities, and even wilder rumors spread that he was facing the death penalty. What was certain was that his laboratory at Southern University of Science and Technology had been closed down. JK was finally photographed on the balcony of an apartment in a hotel on the university campus, where he evidently was living with his wife and children. There were security personnel outside his apartment. Their affiliation and whether they were on hand to keep JK in or to keep others out for his protection were unclear. He continued to have access to the Internet and to email, keeping tabs on news articles about him and communicating with colleagues.

As was to be expected, there were many, many news articles about JK and the gene-edited twins in the weeks following Antonio Regalado's and Marilynn Marchione's initial stories. In the days immediately after JK's Summit presentation, journalists took special note of JK's claim that he had discussed his clinical trial with several American scientists and ethicists and sought out confirmation whether this was true.

Most deeply involved, apparently, was Dr. Michael Deem at Rice University in Houston. JK had specifically acknowledged Deem's contributions to his clinical trial. A quick look at his Rice University website revealed Deem to be a physicist and engineer. It didn't seem that Deem had any special expertise to offer when it came to gene editing of babies. His connection with JK wasn't hard to find—Deem was JK's research advisor when the latter was at graduate school at Rice. JK had included him as a coauthor on many of the manuscripts JK had published after starting his own laboratory in Shenzhen. Was JK's acknowledgment of Deem nothing more than courtesy for a revered mentor? Did Deem have any clue about Lulu and Nana?

He did. In her initial story for the Associated Press, Marchione quoted Deem as saying, "Of course the work occurred. I met the parents. I was there for the informed consent of the parents." Not only did Deem not deny knowing anything about JK's clinical trial, he essentially bragged about his involvement in it. It was no surprise that within hours of the publication of Marchione's article, Rice University launched an investigation.

In interviews later that week, several people including Drs. Matthew Porteus and William Hurlbut at Stanford University and Dr. Mark DeWitt at the University of California, Berkeley, reported that JK had discussed his interest in a clinical trial to target *CCR5* in human embryos and establish pregnancies. He had even mentioned receiving approval from an ethics committee for the trial. Each of them had tried to dissuade JK from going forward with the trial. "I think he was expecting me to be more receptive, and I was very negative," Porteus told the Associated Press. "I was angry at his naivete, I was angry at his recklessness." Plainly their advice was lost on JK. Perhaps taken aback by his confidants' negative reactions, JK kept to himself the news of the actual pregnancy resulting in Lulu and Nana until shortly before the Summit. "I didn't hear from him and assumed he would not proceed," said Porteus. "In retrospect, I could have raised a hue and cry."

Months later, it emerged that at least two other prominent scientists had been in the know all along about JK's activities. Dr. Stephen Quake at Stanford University, who served as JK's research mentor during a year the latter had spent at Stanford after finishing his PhD studies at Rice, had been aware of JK's intentions about gene-edited babies as early as 2016. Quake told *The New York Times* that he had discouraged JK from pursuing the work, but said that he told JK that if he was going to do it, he needed to obtain approval from a local ethics committee. In 2017, JK emailed Quake to let him know that he had received the necessary approvals, and in April 2018 he sent Quake the message: "Good News! The women is pregnant, the genome editing success! The embryo with CCR5 gene edited was transplanted 10 days ago, and today the pregnancy is confirmed!" Quake responded: "Wow, that's quite an achievement! Hopefully she will carry to term …"

In October 2018, Quake learned from JK of a successful birth: "Great news! the baby is born (please keep it in confidential)." JK also made a request: "I want get help from you on how to announce the result, PR and ethics." After Quake was again reassured that ethics approvals were in place, he provided the requested help right up until JK's presentation at the Summit in Hong Kong. When asked by *The New York Times* whether in retrospect he should have done things differently, Quake responded: "Well, hindsight is twenty-twenty. I mean, you could say yes I should have done many other things." Citing his belief that JK had the appropriate ethics approvals, Quake said: "To the extent that it wasn't obvious misconduct, what does a person in my position do? Encourage him to do it right, his research, right? I mean, that's what I believed I was doing."

As reported by the Associated Press, the other scientist, Dr. Craig Mello at the University of Massachusetts Medical School, was rather less supportive of JK's endeavor. Since October 2017, Mello had been serving as a scientific advisor to a company JK had founded in China called Direct Genomics. In April 2018, JK sent Mello an email message almost identical to the one he sent to Quake announcing the establishment of the pregnancy. Mello responded by making clear his disapproval: "I'm glad for you, but I'd rather not be kept in the loop on this. I think this is not a true unmet medical need, and so do not support the use of CRISPR for this indication. You are risking the health of the child you are editing ... I just don't see why you are doing this. I wish your patient the best of luck for a healthy pregnancy." Yet despite his concerns, Mello chose to respect the confidentiality of JK's news.

In one of my own numerous conversations with journalists during the week of the Summit, one of them asked me whether JK had ever reached out to me, whether I had an inkling of what he was up to. I said no. I had not even seen or heard the name He Jiankui before receiving his manuscript from Marchione the previous week.

The journalist's question stuck with me. On Saturday morning, several days after JK's announcement of the twins, I had my first opportunity to reflect on events after a busy week of interviews. I wondered whether I might have interacted with JK without realizing it. I typed in "He Jiankui" in the search bar on the laptop computer on which I did most of my day-to-day work. My stomach dropped when the search function came up with an unexpected hit.

The hit was a manuscript I had received from a prominent scientific journal, *Science Translational Medicine*, a few months earlier. I had been asked to serve as a peer reviewer. This meant my job was to evaluate the manuscript and make one of three recommendations. First option: the manuscript was of such good quality and novelty that it should be published immediately. Second option: the manuscript had flaws, but could be improved with further experimentation; the authors should have the chance to do more work and then send in a revised version of the manuscript. Third option: even with extensive work the manuscript couldn't possibly be improved to the point where it would merit publication in the journal, and so it should be rejected outright.

The title of this manuscript was "Targeted PCSK9 genome editing in embryos by CRISPR-Cas9 system." Given my experience in gene editing and especially my interest in the *PCSK9* gene—I had spent years working on it and published several papers describing the work—it made sense that the journal would ask me to be a peer reviewer. I readily agreed, though I was busy and didn't have much time to spend on the task. At a glance, I saw the author list was a string of Chinese names. None of them matched any gene-editing expert familiar to me.

I was much more interested in the content of the manuscript, especially after seeing this sentence in the abstract: "Here we used CRISPR-Cas9-mediated genome editing to target *PCSK9* in human, monkey and mouse embryos." Indeed, much of the manuscript focused on the use of a particular CRISPR guide RNA—which the authors called sgRNA2—to efficiently inactivate the *PCSK9* gene via NHEJ repair in viable human embryos. There was no question the gene had been inactivated in some of the human embryos. But the authors had also found the majority of the embryos were mosaic. Furthermore, while a search for sgRNA2 off-target effects in the embryos had not turned up anything, the methods used by the authors had been relatively crude and not up to the standards of the gene-editing field.

In all, the work did not strike me as particularly encouraging. So I was taken aback by the authors' conclusion that "the efficacy and safety of our *in vitro* and *in vivo* studies presented here suggest that targeted *PCSK9* genome editing in embryos by CRISPR-Cas9 system provides a potential strategy for the prevention and treatment of familial hypercholesterolemia and coronary heart disease." There was nothing in the manuscript to suggest any human embryos had been used to establish pregnancies. But clearly gene-edited babies had been on the authors' minds. Still, at the time I hadn't put much stock in what I thought was hyperbolic language intended to spice up the manuscript.

After reading the manuscript, I recommended that the journal reject it outright. It was an easy call. The work lacked novelty—going as far back as 2015, several groups had already used CRISPR-Cas9 to edit genes in human embryos. Simply editing another gene—*PCSK9*—which wasn't the focus of any of the earlier studies didn't seem to me to be a genuine scientific advance. It came across as unoriginal, me-too work. I also criticized the inadequate assessment of safety, namely the question of sgRNA2 off-target effects.

In my written review, I also expressed my ethical concerns: "I find it concerning that the authors would so willingly embrace the notion of editing human embryos when there would be no clear benefit to doing so compared to performing somatic gene editing after children are born or, better, after they have reached the age of majority and can give their own consent to the procedure. This is not a situation where newborns will experience high mortality or great suffering and where a reasonable argument could be made for intervening before birth, as early as the embryo stage." My intent was to convey to the authors that they needed to be more judicious in their language. It is common practice for researchers to promote their work by invoking some imagined future in which the work will pay off by helping lots of patients. But I thought the authors' loose talk of someday editing human embryos to treat high cholesterol levels—when there was no real medical reason to do so—wasn't helping their case in trying to get their work published.

In those innocent days in the early fall of 2018, it hadn't occurred to me that the authors might already be rushing ahead to use *PCSK9*-edited human embryos to establish pregnancies.

On the basis of my negative recommendation, as well as feedback from other peer reviewers, the journal decided to reject the *PCSK9* manuscript. Since I never heard anything further about it, and it was just one of dozens of manuscripts I was asked by various journals to review that year, I put it out of my mind. When months later I received JK's manuscript about the *CCR5*-edited twins from Marchione, I had no particular reason to connect it to *PCSK9*. It was only afterward, on that Saturday when I was searching my hard drive, that the connection became clear. The search pulled up the *PCSK9* manuscript. And I was shocked to realize that the senior author of the *PCSK9* manuscript—the last name in the author list—was none other than "Jiankui He" (how JK rendered his name in scientific publications): a name that meant nothing to me a few months earlier, but was now receiving worldwide attention.

With the benefit of hindsight, I took a fresh look at the *PCSK9* manuscript. Another name that meant nothing to me when I first read the manuscript was now instantly recognizable: Michael Deem, who was the next-to-last author. The name of the first author, Feifei Cheng, tugged at my memory. *Where have I seen that name before?* A search of my hard drive with the name turned up nothing besides the *PCSK9* manuscript. Then I thought to search my email. There were multiple hits, dating back to about one year earlier, in late 2017.

The first email was an unsolicited message from Cheng with the subject line "about targeting PCSK9 genome editing in embryos." A PhD graduate student hailing from Southern University of Science and Technology of China—who, I now realized, was a student in JK's laboratory—Cheng had been seeking advice. "Our laboratory are doing some research about targeting PCSK9 genome editing in embryos by CRISPR/Cas9 technology, which might provide a novel insight in the prevent and treatment of familial hypercholesterolemia and cardiovascular disease. Now our results have shown that CRISPR/Cas9 technology can reach a high editing efficiency for PCSK9 gene in human and monkey embryos." After giving a few more details, Cheng asked: "I have read your several papers about targeting PCSK9 genome editing, and know that you have done very good research in this area. So I want to know how you think our research. Do you think it is reasonable and feasible?"

After I responded with a noncommittal message—I didn't have much advice to offer, and I didn't think the *PCSK9* work would add much to what was already known—Cheng replied: "I think our research will illustrate whether targeting PCSK9 genome editing **in embryos, not in adult**, [emphasis Cheng's] is efficient and safe for the first time." Though it didn't explicitly mention pregnancy, this reply seemed to telegraph a motivation to eventually go in that direction. Why else would there be a mention of safety? I wanted no part of it, and I didn't reply in turn.

Shortly afterward, I received another message from Cheng. This one wasn't simply a request for advice, but a request for materials I had created in my own laboratory. "I find that you have constructed BE3-GFP-PC-SK9(Q302) in your research named 'In Vivo Base Editing of PCSK9 (Proprotein Convertase Subtilisin/Kexin Type 9) as a Therapeutic Alternative to Genome Editing.' This is the plasmid that I want to use in my research. So could you give me a little bit of BE3-GFP-PCSK9(Q302) plasmid and its control plasmid? I will pay the delivery cost and try to seek for later cooperation." Cheng was asking for a tool I had made for base editing of *PCSK9*. This tool was only useful to inactivate the human version of the gene, not the monkey or mouse versions. It was clear that Cheng's intended use of the plasmid was to edit human embryos. I left the message unanswered and didn't hear from Cheng again.

As it turned out, Cheng hadn't really needed my advice. The various papers my laboratory had published on *PCSK9* editing were in the scientific literature, available on the Internet for anybody in the world to read. That included JK's team of researchers. As I was taking a second look at JK's *PCSK9* manuscript, I came to a startling realization. The CRISPR guide RNA the authors had used to inactivate *PCSK9* in human embryos, sgRNA2, was identical to a guide RNA I had published in a paper in 2016. I missed this detail when I originally reviewed the paper. My laboratory had worked hard to identify this particular guide RNA and to show that it efficiently and safely inactivates the *PCSK9* gene in human liver cells, making it a potential candidate for an adult therapy. JK hadn't had to spend any extra effort—he just lifted the guide RNA sequence from my paper and applied it to human embryos.

In case there was any doubt that JK had been reading my papers and borrowing liberally from my work, there was another detail that I somehow missed when I first read the *PCSK9* manuscript. JK actually name-checked me, right there in the manuscript: "Of note, Musunuru K et al. used adenovirus to express Cas9 and sgRNA targeted *Pcsk9* in mouse liver, and observed a >50 percent mutagenesis rate of *Pcsk9* with concomitant reduction of plasma PCSK9 and cholesterol levels. Similar results were obtained when they used CRISPR-Cas9 system to target the human *PCSK9* gene in chimeric liver-humanized mice bearing human hepatocytes."

It seemed that all along JK had been pursuing *PCSK9*, a gene-editing target to protect against familial hypercholesterolemia and heart disease, in parallel with his pursuit of *CCR5*, a target to protect against HIV infection. Adding to the evidence, Regalado tracked down documentation on the Chinese Clinical Trial Registry website describing a study with the title "Evaluating the safety of genome editing in abandoned human embryos and in monkey and mouse embryos" and registered under JK's name. It had a retrospective registration date of October 18, 2018, and a backdated start date of April 1, 2017. The study description contained the following language: "In this study, we will use the most popular CRISPR/Cas9 gene-editing technology and its derivative single base mutation technology to carry out exploratory experiments on the abandoned human embryo samples … At present, we have selected the CCR5 and PCSK9 genes as the research targets." There was no mention of establishing pregnancies.

Several months later Preetika Rana reported in *The Wall Street Journal* that JK's original plan for creating the world's first gene-edited babies had been to tackle familial hypercholesterolemia, which meant editing *PCSK9*. It was only after visiting an AIDS village that he had changed his mind and decided to make *CCR5* his first target. Whether he had been genuinely moved by the suffering of HIV patients or whether he felt that society would be more receptive to a treatment that protected against HIV is unclear. Regardless, it appears that he subsequently had misgivings about his choice. As stated in the article in *The Wall Street Journal*: "At times, Dr. He questioned whether he had been too emotional in choosing to target HIV, and should have stuck with familial hypercholesterolemia or picked a different disease, people he consulted say."

Why was JK so interested in *PCSK9* in the first place? Like *CCR5*, it offered the advantage of simplicity. If he could simply turn off the gene—regardless of how it was done, of which mutations were inserted into the gene—there would arguably be a beneficial effect. It would immediately be apparent in any live-born children whether the editing had been successful. Their LDL cholesterol levels would be unusually low. And while there might be controversy about the ethical implications of JK's achievement, there wouldn't be much debate over the scientific premise. After all, three percent of people are naturally born with *PCSK9* mutations; there are drugs on the market that reproduce the effects of the mutations in patients who are part of the other ninety-seven percent; and the drugs provably reduce the risk of heart disease. I certainly hadn't been shy about trumpeting the potential benefits of *PCSK9* editing for adult patients at risk for heart disease, whether in my published papers or in presentations I gave at international conferences or in interviews I gave to the press. How much of that messaging might have rubbed off on JK?

When I discovered my unwelcome connections to JK via our shared interest in the *PCSK9* gene, I felt as sick to my stomach as I had when I first learned about Lulu and Nana two weeks earlier. If events had played out slightly differently, the world's first gene-edited babies would have been *PCSK9*-edited babies rather than *CCR5*-edited babies, using technology directly plucked from my own published research. Even now, it seemed plausible that the second pregnancy JK announced at the Summit involved *PCSK9*-edited embryos rather than *CCR5*-edited embryos. The idea that I might have been complicit in such a dubious deed, however unknowingly and unwillingly, was deeply disturbing.

During the next few months, I had plenty of time to reflect on whether there was anything I could have done to prevent the birth of the gene-edited twins. It would be all too easy to criticize the scientists and bioethicists who were in JK's confidence for not blowing the whistle on him. But would I have acted any differently if I'd been in their position?

Except that I had actually tried to tell others about my concerns. And not just my colleagues—I had tried to tell my own government. In late 2017, soon after I heard from Feifei Cheng in JK's laboratory and had reason to suspect that at least one group of researchers in China had ambitions of creating gene-edited babies, I had the opportunity to brief a group of Congressional staffers via telephone. They wanted to learn about CRISPR, as well as identify experts to testify in person to the U.S. Senate Committee on Health, Education, Labor and Pensions. They were probably hoping to hear about the wonders of CRISPR and how it was going to revolutionize the treatment of disease. Instead, I warned them about the dangers of human embryo editing and the prospect of gene-edited babies in the coming years, most likely in China. It ended up being an awkward conversation, and no invitation to Capitol Hill was forthcoming.

I now wonder whether things might have turned out differently if I had instead shared my concerns in late 2017 with a doggedly determined journalist like Antonio Regalado. Armed with my emails from Cheng, might he have uncovered JK's activities and shone on them a bright light for the whole world to see? Before Lulu's and Nana's parents made the fateful decision to allow JK's team to proceed with the pregnancy?

11

A HISTORIC ETHICAL FIASCO

On January 21, 2019—a little less than two months after JK announced the world's first gene-edited babies—the Xinhua News Agency, China's state-run press agency, reported the results of an official government investigation in Guangdong Province (where Southern University of Science and Technology in the city of Shenzhen is located) into JK's activities. The conclusion, as translated into English by *South China Morning Post*, was that starting in 2016 JK had privately "organised a project team that included foreign staff, which intentionally avoided surveillance and used technology of uncertain safety and effectiveness to perform human embryo gene-editing activity with the purpose of reproduction, which is officially banned in the country." Disavowing any involvement by the Chinese government, the investigators claimed that JK had raised his own funds for the project "in pursuit of personal fame and fortune."

The investigation confirmed that twin baby girls had been born and that a second pregnancy was underway. It also found that JK had forged ethics documents and had evaded a ban in China on HIV-positive parents undergoing assisted reproduction (in vitro fertilization) by substituting HIV-negative blood samples from other people. As translated into English by *The New York Times*, his "behavior seriously violated ethics, scientific research integrity and relevant state regulations causing adverse effects at home and abroad." The head of the investigation team promised JK would "be dealt with seriously according to the law," with the case "handed over to public security organs," and that Guangdong Province would provide medical observation and follow-up care for the babies and the pregnant mother.

In light of the findings of the investigation, Southern University of Science and Technology immediately announced that it had terminated JK's employment at the institution (he had been on unpaid leave since the news of the gene-edited babies had broken).

It wasn't clear which specific Chinese laws, regulations, or guidelines JK had violated. Commentators pointed to a 2003 regulatory document issued by the Ministry of Health with the (translated) title "Technical Norms on Human Assisted Reproductive Technologies." It stated: "The use of genetically manipulated human gametes, zygotes and embryos for the purpose of reproduction is prohibited." (Gametes include sperm cells and egg cells.) But it did not specify any penalties. There were other regulations that, with sufficiently liberal interpretations, JK could be deemed to have breached. In general, these regulations were written long before anybody could have contemplated the use of CRISPR-Cas9 to modify human embryos. In light of these ambiguities, the Chinese government took quick action to deter other local scientists from following in JK's footsteps. The National Health Commission drafted new gene-editing regulations with severe penalties, and a draft of the country's updated civil code included new protections for subjects of gene-editing research.

Regardless of whether JK's actions actually contravened Chinese law, there was a widespread sense that he'd flouted international norms. An in-depth examination of the circumstances that resulted in the birth of the gene-edited twins shows that JK violated numerous bedrock principles of ethical medical research. Indeed, JK's conduct stands out as an instructive example of how one should **not** carry out medical research, in almost every respect.

At every institution at which I have trained or worked since graduating from high school, I have had to undergo human subjects research training every few years. In other words, learn and re-learn how to do medical research involving human beings in a responsible, ethical manner. The training typically has involved a combination of online coursework—a mix of documents to read, videos to watch, and multiple-choice quizzes to pass—and meetings in small groups in classrooms to discuss case studies. Since the subject material doesn't change much, if at all, from year to year, after doing the training a few times it comes across as repetitive and boring. In most researchers' eyes, I suspect, the training is simply a box to be checked and something to get through as quickly and painlessly as possible.

JK's misadventures with gene editing offer a strong argument why human subjects research training is perhaps the most important education any medical researcher ever receives.

The training invariably starts by citing the atrocities committed by Nazi Germany on civilians and prisoners of war in concentration camps in the name of medical research. The human experimentation involved deliberate head injuries; removal of body parts; freezing; incendiary bombs; high altitude conditions; deprivation of all food except seawater; poisons; pathogens; and experimental drugs and vaccines against those pathogens. Often the subjects were killed afterward so the scientists could assess the effects of the experiments on the human body. In a particularly odious group of experiments, the infamous Josef Mengele (nicknamed the Angel of Death) exploited fifteen hundred sets of twins. In many cases, he experimented on one twin and spared the other, so that he could directly compare the bodies of the twins—sometimes after executing both twins.

After World War II, as part of the Nuremberg trials, twenty-three medical doctors and Nazi officials were tried for war crimes and crimes against humanity in relation to the medical experiments performed without the subjects' consent. In this so-called Doctors' Trial, seven defendants received death sentences and nine received prison sentences. The verdict of the trial outlined ten principles of "permissible medical experiments" that later came to be known as the Nuremberg Code. Woven into these principles were the concepts of informed consent, lack of coercion, potential for benefit, and minimization of harm, as well as the requirement that experiments be conducted only by scientifically qualified persons. The Nuremberg Code has influenced all subsequent attempts to codify ethical principles governing medical research, most notably the Declaration of Helsinki first promulgated by the World Medical Association in 1964.

The Nuremberg Code, the Declaration of Helsinki, and other such documents don't carry the force of international law. Nonetheless, the general principles enunciated in these documents have been incorporated into the laws of many nations, including China. As such, they're the closest thing to universal principles of ethical medical research that we're likely to have for the foreseeable future. That these principles need to be continually taught and refreshed in the minds of researchers should never be in doubt. Liberal democracies such as the United States are not immune to gross ethical violations at the government level.

In the Tuskegee Study of Untreated Syphilis in the African American, run by the U.S. Public Health Service starting in 1932, several hundred African American men with syphilis were studied for four decades. Penicillin proved to be an effective treatment for syphilis in the 1940s, after the Tuskegee Study had begun. Yet the researchers never told the subjects that they had syphilis. Worse, the researchers went out of their way to prevent the subjects from receiving penicillin, since their goal was to see how untreated syphilis infections progressed over time. There was no possibility of informed consent by the subjects, nor did the researchers act to minimize harm.

The Tuskegee Study ended in 1972 only after a whistleblower shared details of the study with *The Washington Star* and *The New York Times*, making it front page news. By that time, more than a quarter of the subjects had died as a result of their untreated syphilis, after having passed the infection to dozens of their wives and children. It wasn't until twenty-five years later that President Bill Clinton formally apologized to the Tuskegee victims on behalf of the U.S. government.

One consequence of the Tuskegee scandal was the formation of the U.S. National Commission for the Protection of Human Subjects of Biomedical and Behavioral Research. In 1978, the Commission issued *The Belmont Report*, which has served as the source of ethical principles and guidelines for medical research in the United States ever since. Influenced by previous standards such as the Nuremberg Code and the Declaration of Helsinki, *The Belmont Report* laid out three basic ethical principles— respect for persons, beneficence, and justice—and three applications of those principles—informed consent, assessment of risks and benefits, and selection of subjects.

Much of the human subjects research training at U.S. institutions centers on a discussion of *The Belmont Report* and its implications for clinical trials performed by U.S. researchers. One consequence of *The Belmont Report* is that medical research funded by the U.S. federal government requires approval by an ethics committee known as an Institutional Review Board (IRB). Fundamentally, the IRB's role is to safeguard the rights and welfare of subjects involved in medical research. The IRB is charged with reviewing a proposed research project and assessing whether it conforms to the ethical principles and applications laid out in *The Belmont Report*. If not, the IRB will reject the project, and it can insist on substantial changes before approving the project. The IRB can also terminate an ongoing project if there are ethical lapses. U.S. law, specifically Title 45 Code of Federal Regulations Part 46, lays out all the parameters for how an IRB should operate—the IRB's responsibilities, its powers, who can serve as an IRB member, and so forth.

Though *The Belmont Report* might not be required reading outside of the United States, many countries around the world have enshrined the same ethical principles and applications in their laws. In China, the National Health Commission has laid out the operating procedures for research ethics committees (equivalent to IRBs) in its Guidelines on Ethical Review of Biomedical Research Involving Human Subjects and in its Management Guidelines for Conducting Clinical Research at Medical/ Health Institutions (translated titles). How rigorously these guidelines are enforced at individual Chinese medical institutions is unclear.

As we shall see, JK's team was guilty of violating all of the aforementioned ethical principles. Perhaps this can be blamed on the ignorance of the team's leaders. But that doesn't really hold water. JK obtained a PhD at Rice University and spent a year doing postdoctoral work at Stanford University. It's hard to believe that he wasn't required to take human subjects research training at some point during his training. Even more so for Dr. Michael Deem, JK's former PhD advisor and later collaborator on JK's gene-editing work who claimed "I was there for the informed consent of the parents"—he was a professor of bioengineering at Rice for many years. One possible defense is that neither JK nor Deem was ever involved in medical research involving human beings while at Rice or Stanford, and so neither would have needed to take human subjects research training. But if that's the case, what qualified JK to oversee a clinical trial involving a highly experimental technology with lifelong consequences for the subjects involved?

Let's consider all of the ways in which JK's efforts to create the world's first gene-edited babies breached widely accepted principles of medical ethics.

Respect for persons. *The Belmont Report* states: "Respect for persons incorporates at least two basic ethical convictions: first, that individuals should be treated as autonomous agents, and second, that persons with diminished autonomy are entitled to protection." JK's clinical trial involved two sets of individuals. First, the prospective parents, especially the mothers who would have to bear the pregnancies. Second, the unborn descendants who would bear the consequences of the gene editing. These descendants of course include the people arising from the edited embryos, such as Lulu and Nana, but also include future generations who might inherit the edits, such as Lulu's and Nana's children. The degree to which the parents in the clinical trial were treated as autonomous should be judged by the integrity of the informed consent process—which, as explained below, was greatly lacking. The unborn descendants, of course, had zero autonomy since they had yet to come into existence.

There is ample precedent for parents giving consent on behalf of their child for medical research, on account of the latter's diminished autonomy. Nonetheless, the bar for accepting a child into a study should be much higher than for an adult with full autonomy. From *The Belmont Report*: "Some persons are in need of extensive protection, even to the point of excluding them from activities which may harm them ... The extent of protection afforded should depend upon the risk of harm and the likelihood of benefit."

Beneficence. *The Belmont Report* states: "Persons are treated in an ethical manner not only by respecting their decisions and protecting them from harm, but also by making efforts to secure their well-being ... Two general rules have been formulated as complementary expressions of beneficent actions in this sense: (1) do not harm and (2) maximize possible benefits and minimize possible harms." The first rule, "do no harm," is quite familiar to students training to become physicians, tied as it is to the Hippocratic Oath that traditionally has served as a guide to the conduct of medical practitioners. This rule is similar to the ethical principle of non-maleficence, discussed in the next point.

With respect to maximizing the possible benefits to the research subjects, JK's clinical trial fell woefully short. For Nana, who bears two mutated copies of the *CCR5* gene in her body (putting aside the possibility of mosaicism), the potential benefit is lifetime resistance to HIV infection. Of course, there's reason to doubt that her resistance extends to all HIV strains, since individuals born with two copies of the *CCR5* Δ32 mutation aren't protected against all strains. Even so, will Nana truly benefit from her editing? Her father is HIV-positive but has the infection suppressed with medical treatment, so the chance of him passing the infection to a child is essentially zero. Nana's lifetime risk of being exposed to HIV is no different from any of her peers. Any of her peers who became infected with HIV, despite reasonable precautions, would be able to take medications to suppress the virus and would have very little chance of progressing to AIDS and dying from it. And this assumes that no cure for HIV will become available within Nana's lifetime. Has Nana actually benefited in any meaningful way compared to her peers, or compared to a version of herself who didn't have the edits? It doesn't seem so.

Lulu, who supposedly bears only one mutated copy of the *CCR5* gene in her body, wouldn't experience the same resistance to HIV as her sister. Her chance of becoming infected with HIV is about the same as any of her peers. She has even less to gain from her editing.

It's hard to make a compelling case that either Nana or Lulu received much in the way of benefit from JK's clinical trial. But there is another argument that could be made, which is that humanity will benefit from the clinical trial. Nana and Lulu showed that it was possible to edit human embryos and establish pregnancies resulting in (apparently) healthy live-born babies. No matter that Nana and Lulu didn't personally benefit in a medical sense. They have paved the way for many children in the future to be spared from genetic diseases—millions of children, if JK's YouTube propaganda is to be believed—which could add up to a very large benefit indeed.

Arguments like this one ignore the fact that Nana and Lulu will bear substantial risks for the rest of their lives. Theoretical benefits to people in the future cannot on their own justify a clinical trial. The possibility of harm to the research subjects is an even more important consideration.

Non-maleficence. The potential harms to Nana, Lulu, and any other children born as a result of JK's clinical trial are numerous.

First, gene-editing technology is nowhere close to being perfected. The outcomes of its use can't be fully controlled or predicted. Nana and Lulu were born prematurely, after about seven months of pregnancy— was this because of their embryos' exposure to CRISPR-Cas9? Because of mosaicism, Nana and Lulu are likely to have bodies that are patchworks of edited cells, whether edits in the *CCR5* gene or off-target edits. The health consequences of this mosaicism are unknown.

Second, there are unintended consequences of the intended editing to consider. The available evidence suggests that the *CCR5* edits intended to make Nana and Lulu resistant to HIV will make them more vulnerable to other viral infections: West Nile virus, tick-borne encephalitis virus, and, of greatest concern, flu viruses. If either twin were to pick up a flu infection, it is substantially more likely to be serious and even fatal. JK was well aware of this possibility when he carried out his clinical trial.

Third, there are the consequences of unintended off-target editing. There might be serious health consequences such as cancer or heart disease even if only a small proportion of the cells in the body have off-target mutations. Worse, if one of the twins were to develop, say, childhood cancer, it would be impossible to know for sure whether it was the result of the CRISPR-Cas9 editing or simply the kind of bad luck that can strike any child.

Fourth, the risks are inherent not just to Nana and Lulu but possibly to future generations. If the original editing resulted in harmful mutations in their cells, they could pass on the mutations to their own children. It might be that the only way to ensure their children would be healthy would be for them to use in vitro fertilization and have the embryos probed to make sure they carry no harmful mutations. Given the risks, is it possible that the twins might actually be forced by their government to use in vitro fertilization and not be permitted to conceive naturally if they wish to have children?

Fifth, from the perspective of the dignity of human life, the twins were treated by JK's team not as patients—there was no disease that was cured, and there was no unmet medical need—but primarily as subjects of human experimentation. Will they continue to be treated that way for the rest of their lives? Required to submit to frequent medical examinations and testing? Will their own children be treated that way too?

Sixth, the twins might be perceived in negative ways by their family, their peers, their society—and by themselves. What will it mean to them that they were the first to be subjected to an experimental medical procedure, for no particularly good medical reason? Will it somehow undermine their self-perception? Will they be shunned by their peers and potential partners? Will their privacy be compromised? On the flip side, will it impermissibly undermine the twins' autonomy if the knowledge that they were edited as embryos is withheld from them?

Justice. *The Belmont Report* asks: "Who ought to receive the benefits of research and bear its burdens? This is a question of justice, in the sense of 'fairness in distribution' or 'what is deserved.'" Citing both the Nazi concentration camps and the Tuskegee Study as egregious examples of injustice, *The Belmont Report* asserts that "the selection of research subjects needs to be scrutinized in order to determine whether some classes (e.g., welfare patients, particular racial and ethnic minorities, or persons confined to institutions) are being systematically selected simply because of their easy availability, their compromised position, or their manipulability, rather than for reasons directly related to the problem being studied."

With JK's clinical trial, the case for injustice is not as clear-cut as for the violations of other ethical principles. Nonetheless, JK's choice to restrict his clinical trial to HIV-positive fathers (and HIV-negative mothers) as study participants, where there was essentially no chance of HIV transmission to their children, seems problematic. There was no medical reason to limit the trial to HIV-positive fathers. But with the social stigma of being HIV-positive in China and, especially, with HIV-positive parents being banned from undergoing assisted reproduction, the door was open to exploitation of a class of persons. Namely, infertile HIV-positive parents who were desperate for children and had no other access to in vitro fertilization except through JK's clinical trial. Why didn't JK open his trial to all couples who were interested in having children resistant to HIV? Did he feel it would be easier to convince desperate HIV-positive fathers to allow their unborn children to be subjected to the risks of an experimental medical procedure?

One of JK's comments during his Summit presentation only reinforces the notion that he was exploiting the study participants. "And also for this specific case, I feel proud, actually. I feel proudest, because [the father] thought that he lost hope for the life. But when the babies were born, with this protection, he sent a message at their birth saying I will work hard, earn money, and take care of his two daughters and his wife ..." The father doesn't sound like he's specifically grateful that his children might be protected against HIV. He sounds like someone who's grateful to have children at all, who would have been just as happy if he'd been given two healthy children and gene editing had never been in the picture.

Informed consent. *The Belmont Report* states: "Respect for persons requires that subjects, to the degree that they are capable, be given the opportunity to choose what shall or shall not happen to them. This opportunity is provided when adequate standards for informed consent are satisfied." It goes on to say that the consent process has three elements— information, comprehension, and voluntariness. Are the potential research subjects provided with enough information, including a full accounting of the benefits and risks of participating in the study, to make an informed decision? Do they fully understand the information provided to them? And are they voluntarily giving consent to participate in the study, free of coercion (overt threat of harm if they don't agree to participate), and free of undue influence (offer of an excessive, unwarranted, inappropriate, or improper reward if they agree to participate)?

After making his initial announcement about Nana and Lulu, JK posted the informed consent document used for his clinical trial on his laboratory website, so there's not much ambiguity about how he approached the consent process. The document mentions only two benefits to study participants: "This research project will likely help you produce HIV-resistant infants" and "The project team purchases Ping An Group's Anxingbao insurance for babies born."

The document lists several potential harms, mostly related to the routine process of assisted reproduction:

- Ovarian hyperstimulation syndrome and other adverse effects of the drug treatment used to prime the mother to produce more mature eggs than usual.

- Anesthesia risk, surgical complications, bleeding, or infection as a result of the harvesting of the eggs from the mother.

- The possibility that in vitro fertilization will fail to produce viable embryos.

- The possibility "that some embryos may not have anti-AIDs ability."

- The possibility of in vitro fertilization transmitting HIV to the baby, since the father is HIV-positive.

- Birth defects and common genetic diseases that "belong to the scope of natural risk of natural reproduction."

All well and good—these are the sorts of hazards that are supposed to be described as part of the informed consent process—but they are largely the same hazards faced by any couple undergoing assisted reproduction. When it comes to the one aspect of the protocol that's experimental, the editing of the embryos, the document lists only one possible risk: "The primary risk of gene editing (DNA-targeted CRISPR-Cas9 endonuclease) is the off-target effect of generating extra DNA mutations at sites other than the intended target. This is due to that the technique can cause nonspecific cleavage, resulting in mutations in non-targeted genomic sites." There's no further explanation of what this could mean for the health of a baby. Instead, there is a disclaimer that "this project team is not responsible for the risk of off-target which is beyond the risk consequences of the existing medical science and technology."

The informed consent document is extraordinary in that it's full of disclaimers and assertions of rights on the part of the research team. It reads like a contract that favors the researchers more than the study participants—surely not what was envisioned by the drafters of the Nuremberg Code, the Declaration of Helsinki, or *The Belmont Report*.

- "The rights and obligations in the testing shall be based on the contract between you and the medical institution."

- "In case of any disputes over rights and obligations during the project period between you and the medical institution, the contract signed shall prevail, and the project team is not responsible for this."

- "It is normal if the infants do not have the capacity of natural Immunity to AIDS. The project team does not assume legal responsibility in this situation."

- "The risk [of transmission of HIV to the baby] is **not** [emphasis JK's] caused by this project, and this project team will not take responsibility."

The document outlines publicity rights:

- "Regarding the qualitative characterization of the project results, only the project team has the right of final interpretation and announcement to the public. Then you have **no** [emphasis JK's] right to explain and have **no** [emphasis JK's] right to announce the project or result information without permission. Violation of this will dealt as breach of contract and the volunteers need compensate for the damages (The specifics are defined in the liquidated damages cooperation agreement)."

- "Baby's photo on the day of birth will be kept by the project team. The project team has the portrait right of the infant and can make it open to the public."

- "Regarding the project results, only the project team has the right of final explanation and announcement to the public. The volunteers have no right to explain, publish, or announce project related information without permission."

The document also includes a confidentiality clause: "For the project team's trade secrets, you hereby agree: (1) You strictly observe the secrets of the project team and take all the security measures and systems to protect the secret; (2) You cannot disclose any commercial secrets to any third party; (3) You shall not use the secret at any time except for the purpose of fulfilling the contract with the project team; (4) You can not copy or use the secret through reverse engineering."

Most appalling of all: "After the embryo implantation in the first cycle of IVF until 28 days post-birth of the baby, if you decide to leave the study due to other reasons than the ones listed in Items 3 and 4 above, you will need to pay back all the costs that the project team has paid for you. If the payment is not received within 10 calendar days from the issuance of the notification of violation by the project team, another 100,000 RMB [roughly $15,000] of fine will be charged." A key element of voluntariness is that research subjects can withdraw from a study at any time, for any reason, without consequence. The threat of a large fine exceeding the annual average salary in China is coercion, plain and simple.

Amidst all of the legal language in the informed consent document, there is little description of gene-editing technology, its benefits and harms, and how it might affect the health of a human being. Certainly not enough to ensure that research participants have the necessary information, much less an adequate level of comprehension of that information, to be able to give truly informed consent. At the Summit, JK claimed to have spent one hour and ten minutes going through the whole informed consent document "line by line, paragraph by paragraph" with each set of parents. Perhaps he spent some of that time talking about things that weren't in the document. It is possible he was able to fully convey the nuances and intricacies of gene editing—concepts like DNA cleavage, off-target effects, and mosaicism—to parents who likely had little prior knowledge of genetics. But it stretches credulity.

At the Summit, JK stated that "I read guidelines from the [U.S. National Institutes of Health] on informed consent when we drafted the informed consent." He clearly didn't read the guidelines carefully enough.

Assessment of risks and benefits. *The Belmont Report* states: "It is commonly said that benefits and risks must be 'balanced' and shown to be 'in a favorable ratio.'" Sometimes the determination of whether there's "a favorable ratio" is a judgment call on the part of the IRB or research ethics committee. Nonetheless, we have already seen that the list of potential benefits to the subjects of JK's clinical trial was short, and the list of potential risks was long. There's no reasonable argument to be made that the risks didn't greatly outweigh the benefits.

Even more concerning: for a cutting-edge technology like gene editing that's still very much a work in progress, there are quite possibly risks that remain to be discovered. This makes it even more difficult to judge whether there's "a favorable ratio" of benefits and risks. In such situations, the prudent course of action would be to delay the clinical trial to allow more time for the technology to be studied and the full extent of the risks determined. Why was JK in such a rush to carry out his clinical trial despite the uncertainties about the safety of gene editing? Was the desire to be the first in the world to create gene-edited babies so overwhelming?

A corollary is that if the risks of gene editing aren't well understood by gene-editing researchers, there's certainly no way the risks could be well understood by research subjects, which means that no consent obtained from the participants in JK's clinical trial could be said to be truly informed.

Selection of subjects. *The Belmont Report* states: "Individual justice in the selection of subjects would require that researchers exhibit fairness: thus, they should not offer potentially beneficial research on to some patients who are in their favor or select only 'undesirable' persons for risky research." As already discussed, the choice to restrict to HIV-positive fathers in China is a concerning one, both because of the lack of unmet medical need (there's no particular risk of an HIV-positive father passing the virus to his child) and because of the possibility of exploitation of a vulnerable class of persons (providing the only means for infertile HIV-positive parents to have children). JK's clinical trial might have been slightly more credible if it had been restricted to HIV-positive mothers instead. While there still would have been the concern for exploitation, it's well established that an HIV-positive mother can pass the virus to her child during pregnancy and especially during childbirth. Embryo editing to achieve HIV resistance in the unborn child could reduce that risk. But so too could conventional medical therapy to treat the mother's infection.

Scientific qualifications. *The Belmont Report* doesn't say anything about the qualifications needed in order for researchers to oversee a clinical trial. But the Nuremberg Code has the following as one of its ten principles: "The experiment should be conducted only by scientifically qualified persons. The highest degree of skill and care should be required through all stages of the experiment of those who conduct or engage in the experiment."

JK wasn't a doctor and had no medical training. Rather, he was a physicist who crossed over into biological research. Prior to starting the clinical trial that resulted in Nana and Lulu, he had no experience or formal training in running clinical trials, much less obtaining informed consent from potential research subjects. He had published just one paper on CRISPR, back in 2010 before it had ever been used for human gene editing. He had no notable background in gene editing. My analysis of JK's work suggested to me that JK probably didn't even know how to read chromatograms properly—which, if true, is a startling deficiency for someone professing to be an expert in DNA sequencing and gene editing.

It is hard to believe that anybody who was fully aware of JK's lack of medical and scientific qualifications would want him doing experiments on their children.

Review by a research ethics committee. The notion that JK's clinical trial—with all of its ethical flaws—was somehow approved by a research ethics committee is disturbing enough. The news that the Chinese government's investigation concluded that JK forged ethical documents is even more alarming. JK posted a document with the (translated) title "Medical Ethics Approval Application Form HarMoniCare Shenzhen Women's and Children's Hospital" on the Chinese Clinical Trial Registry website, attached to the registration of his clinical trial. The document appears to have the signatures of the seven members of the hospital's ethics committee, along with the official seal of the committee's chairperson. A hospital administrator, Lin Zhitong, was quoted in Marilynn Marchione's article for the Associated Press that first reported the existence of the gene-edited twins: "We think this is ethical." But during his Summit presentation, when asked how many people reviewed his informed consent document, JK replied "about four people." After the births of Nana and Lulu became worldwide news, the hospital denied any connection to the clinical trial and asserted that the signed approval document in question had been falsified. It's hard to know whom to believe.

JK set out to make history. And so he did, though surely not in the way he intended. JK's clinical trial stands as the biggest medical ethics fiasco of the twenty-first century. Some commentators have gone so far as to liken it to the Nazi concentration camps and the Tuskegee Study (though equating

JK's actions to those of Josef Mengele seems excessive). It wouldn't be surprising if the story of He Jiankui becomes part of the required reading for human subjects research training for future generations of scientists—as a textbook case of all the different ways one can violate the ethical principles of medical research.

In what can only be considered a colossal irony, before the news about the gene-edited babies publicly broke, JK had written a manuscript titled "Draft ethical principles for therapeutic assisted reproductive technologies." Clearly it was intended to lay the groundwork for his announcement about Nana and Lulu. (Oddly enough, one of his co-authors was his American publicist.) JK proposed five core principles as a "first draft of an ethical foundation" for gene editing in human embryos: "mercy for families in need;" "only for serious disease, never vanity;" "respect a child's autonomy;" "genes do not define you;" and "everyone deserves freedom from genetic disease."

The CRISPR Journal, a bona fide scientific journal, accepted JK's ethics manuscript for publication. In truly unfortunate timing, the journal released it the day after JK announced the birth of Nana and Lulu, as his news was being met with widespread condemnation. The reaction to JK's paper from many observers was derision.

It wasn't long before *The CRISPR Journal* retracted JK's paper and expunged it from the scientific literature.

12

THE CRISPR GENERATION

The first members of the CRISPR generation have been born. And more are on the way. It's inevitable.

There's been much talk within the biomedical community about a global moratorium on the editing of human embryos to make genetically modified babies. The word moratorium denotes a temporary ban; eventually it would come to an end. (Surprisingly few commentators have called for a permanent ban.) Even in countries like the United States where laws and regulations currently make it virtually impossible to legally use edited embryos to establish pregnancies, it's hard to believe that things won't eventually change, whether it's five years, ten years, fifty years, or one hundred years in the future. So we had better start thinking hard about what the CRISPR generation will look like.

Putting aside any ethical or legal considerations, why might parents in the future choose to pursue gene editing on behalf of their unborn children? There are three reasons.

The first reason to perform human embryo editing would be the prevention of a grievous genetic disease in a child, where the probability of the child having the disease would otherwise be close to one hundred percent. The goal would be to spare a lifetime of suffering. Well-known diseases like sickle cell disease and cystic fibrosis that affect children from a young age would be in this category. There are a variety of even more rare, less-known genetic diseases that are just as debilitating, if not more so, that would also fit in this category. The common factor among these diseases is that they're driven largely by genetics. For some of these diseases, one mutant copy of the responsible gene pretty much guarantees the disease. (In genetics parlance, these are called dominant disorders.) For others, two mutant copies of the gene are needed in order to have the disease, and having the two bad copies makes the disease almost certain. (These are called recessive disorders.) The only permanent cure for any of these diseases would be a genetic cure.

For some of these diseases, genetic cures are already in development. For example, several companies are planning clinical trials with genetic therapies that could someday be given to kids with sickle cell disease. But these therapies are intended for use after the kids are born. One might argue, why wait until the kids are born and already starting to suffer? Wouldn't it be easier to intervene at the earliest possible time, at the embryo stage, and prevent the suffering altogether? A similar argument based on economics might say that it would be much cheaper to edit a single-cell zygote than to try to fix the whole body of a child.

These arguments have at least two problems. First, making fixes in embryos presupposes that it's already known that the embryos have disease-causing mutations. This would require the parents to know that they have mutations that could be passed on to their children. Right now, in most cases it comes as a surprise to parents when their children turn out to have grievous genetic disorders. The parents never suspected that they had faulty copies of the responsible genes in their own genomes. This situation will change in the coming years, though, as more and more people undergo exome or genome sequencing either for medical reasons or because they're simply curious about what's in their DNA.

The second issue is that editing of embryos requires in vitro fertilization to make the embryos in the first place. Why bother with editing of embryos when it would be easier to screen through the various embryos? Simply identify the ones that do not have the disease-causing mutations, and use those embryos to establish pregnancies. Those children will be safe. Some people object to screening of embryos because it means that invariably some embryos will be discarded, tantamount to the destruction of unborn human life. But gene editing would also result in some discarded embryos due to a lack of the desired edits, the presence of off-target edits, and mosaicism. The same objection would apply.

Let's illustrate the relative merits of screening and gene editing with the example of sickle cell disease, a recessive disorder. In order for a person to have sickle cell disease, there must be two mutant copies of the *HBB* gene, one inherited from the mother, the other from the father. Because of this, we know that each of the parents must have at least one mutant *HBB* copy. Let's say that neither parent has sickle cell disease, which means that neither has two mutant *HBB* copies, since that would definitely result in disease.

If the two prospective parents wished to have a biological child guaranteed to be free of sickle cell disease, how could they go about doing it? If they proceed with natural reproduction, there's a one-in-four chance of any child having the disease. Each parent has a fifty percent chance of passing a mutant copy to the child. So the probability of the child inheriting two mutant copies is fifty percent multiplied by fifty percent, so twenty-five percent. The odds are against the child being sick, but it's far from a guarantee. The parents could instead opt for in vitro fertilization, which results in some number of zygotes being made from their egg cells and sperm cells. The zygotes are grown into blastocysts, followed by pre-implantation genetic diagnosis. This is the standard procedure in which three to five cells are removed from each blastocyst with two to three hundred cells and analyzed for the presence of mutations (similar to how JK's team assessed Lulu's and Nana's embryos before establishing the pregnancy).

We would expect only twenty-five percent of this couple's embryos to have two mutant *HBB* copies. Those embryos would be avoided. On the flip side, twenty-five percent of the embryos would have two normal *HBB* copies. In choosing these embryos for the pregnancy, the parents would ensure not only that their child is free of the disease, but also that the child doesn't carry any mutant *HBB* copies that could be passed to the next generation. Any grandchildren would be safe too.

Would there ever be any reason for editing, then? In vitro fertilization is a chancy procedure that often fails to produce viable embryos. Our couple might undergo several cycles of in vitro fertilization and only end up with a few embryos. What if they were very unlucky and those few embryos all had two mutant *HBB* copies? Being able to edit those embryos and fix at least one of the mutant *HBB* copies might be the only way for them to have a healthy biological child. Or so the argument goes, though it ignores the fact that gene editing to correct mutations is also very chancy, at least with today's technology.

There is another, more realistic scenario to consider. What if both the mother and father have sickle cell disease? This would mean that both have two mutant *HBB* copies. Each would have a one hundred percent chance of passing a mutant *HBB* copy to a child. Put another way, all of their embryos would carry two mutant *HBB* copies, and the resulting children would all have sickle cell disease. There is no possibility of screening embryos to find one that would ensure a healthy child. Here the couple's only option would be embryo editing.

This same scenario applies to any pair of prospective parents who both have the same recessive disease. There is no way for them to have a biological child who's free of their disease without some sort of genetic intervention. How realistic is this scenario? It might have been unheard of even just a generation ago. But now medical advances make it possible for patients with grievous genetic disorders to survive to childbearing age, and

Internet-enabled social networks make it easier for a woman and a man with the same rare disease to meet and forge a romantic connection.

There is another group of people for whom there's no possibility of having a healthy biological child without a genetic intervention—those who have two mutant copies of a gene responsible for a dominant disorder. Just one mutant copy is enough to cause disease. One would have to be truly unlucky to have two copies, though it might not result in disease that's any worse than that experienced by somebody with one copy. It has important implications for childbearing, though. Even if the other parent has normal copies of the gene, every embryo and every resulting child will inherit one mutant copy from the parent with the disease. And so every child will have the disease. Embryo editing to correct the mutant copy might be the only way for a biological child to be healthy.

There might not be many couples who share the same devastating recessive disorder, or individuals with a double dose of dominant mutations, who are seeking to have children. Possibly they number just a few thousand worldwide. Some commentators have pointed out that modern medicine is full of examples where physicians and researchers have gone to extraordinary lengths to relieve the suffering of a few people, or even just one person. That is reason enough to give serious consideration to human embryo editing, despite the scientific and ethical hazards it would entail if it were to become broadly available to society.

Other commentators have asked whether it is worth opening Pandora's box to help such a tiny number of people. They point out that there is an unreasonable presumption to a right to a biological child who shares one's genes. There are other options for parenthood. Many couples, whether infertile or not, choose to adopt children and love them as much as they would biological children. If there is a personal imperative that there must be a sharing of genes with a child, it's still not necessary to turn to embryo editing. One could use sperm and eggs from one parent and from a healthy donor for in vitro fertilization—in the same way many same-sex couples do—so that at least one parent has a biological connection. It would be even better if the donor is a family member, so that both parents have the connection to the child.

A medical colleague of mine recently consulted me about a patient with hypertrophic cardiomyopathy who, upon genetic testing, was found to have two mutant copies of the responsible gene, *MYBPC3*. Because hypertrophic cardiomyopathy is a dominant disorder, the patient is appropriately concerned that any biological child of hers will suffer in the same way that she has from her disease. The question was whether embryo editing would allow her to make sure that her future child would have no predisposition for hypertrophic cardiomyopathy. My answer was yes, but that there is no possibility of embryo editing at the present time. No matter—the patient is considering having her eggs frozen now, on the chance that someday in the future, embryo editing will be safe and legal for patients like her.

The second reason to perform human embryo editing would be to significantly reduce the risk of a child having a serious disease in her lifetime. This might involve common afflictions like heart disease, Alzheimer's disease, and breast cancer. These conditions aren't purely genetic in nature, but they do have genetic components. Heart disease is extremely common—one in two adult men and one in three adult women in the United States experience at least one heart attack in their lifetimes. While many people now survive heart attacks due to better treatments, it remains the leading cause of death worldwide. There are many things people can do to reduce their risk of heart disease, such as exercising, eating a healthy diet, maintaining an ideal body weight, and not smoking. But these measures will not eliminate the risk. At best, they might cut the risk in half. Editing of a gene like *PCSK9* would permanently reduce the amount of cholesterol in the blood and further reduce the risk.

An average man might start at a baseline heart attack risk of fifty percent, but might live a healthy lifestyle and reduce it to twenty-five percent; if his embryo had been edited by his parents to turn off *PCSK9*, his actual risk would be even lower, perhaps ten percent. Alternatively, the same man might have indulged in a hedonistic lifestyle for decades and increased his baseline risk to seventy-five percent, but with editing of his embryo his actual risk could still be better than average, more like thirty percent. (This puts aside the question of whether editing of *PCSK9* as an embryo would offer any advantage over editing of *PCSK9* in the liver during adulthood.) Embryo editing wouldn't ever be able to reduce the risk of heart attack to nothing. Still, parents might find it attractive to tilt the odds in their child's favor even if there's no history of heart disease in the family.

Alzheimer's disease is another example where editing could partially reduce the risk, even if it couldn't reduce the risk to zero. Alzheimer's disease is the most common cause of dementia and is irreversible. There's no proven treatment or behavior that prevents the disease or even slows down its progression. But it's clear that genetics plays a strong role, with numerous genes involved. One gene in particular, *APOE*, seems to have a large influence. There are different versions of *APOE* spread throughout the population. e2, e3, and e4 are the names of the most common versions. It is well established that having one copy of e4 moderately increases one's risk of developing Alzheimer's disease during the lifetime. Having two copies of e4 dramatically increases the risk of disease, though that risk is still far from one hundred percent. To put it another way, many people with two copies of e4 don't develop Alzheimer's disease, and many people with zero copies of e4 still develop disease.

With embryo editing, it's possible to convert e4 copies of the *APOE* gene into e3 copies. Because the entire body of the resulting child will now have more favorable versions of *APOE*, there should be substantially reduced risk of Alzheimer's disease later in life. (Compare embryo editing to trying to change the gene throughout the brain after the child is born—the latter is much more technically challenging.) The risk won't be zero. Embryo editing can't guarantee that the child will never develop Alzheimer's disease. But it's a way to favorably stack the odds. It's not hard to imagine some parents who themselves each have two *APOE* e4 copies wanting to do all they can to protect their children from someday suffering from dementia.

Breast cancer is yet another complex disease where many genes and environmental factors play a role. Nonetheless, it's well established that having a mutation in the *BRCA1* or *BRCA2* gene can substantially increase the risk of a woman (or man) developing breast cancer. Some women go to extraordinary lengths to avoid breast cancer if they discover they have a mutation in one of these genes. In a well-publicized example, the actor Angelina Jolie decided to undergo a preventive double mastectomy (surgical removal of both breasts) after her mother died at age 56 from breast cancer and after Jolie herself was found to have a *BRCA1* mutation and was told by her doctors that she had an eighty-seven percent chance of getting breast cancer in the future. So it's not at all implausible that parents with a strong family history of breast cancer and with a personal *BRCA1* or *BRCA2* mutation might choose to edit their embryos to remove the mutation and potentially spare their child from getting cancer or having to make the choice that Jolie did.

Coronary artery disease, Alzheimer's disease, and breast cancer are quite different from sickle cell disease and cystic fibrosis in multiple ways. The former are common diseases that affect large proportions of the general population; the latter are relatively rare. The former typically occur in adults, especially older adults; the latter cause suffering from the time of childhood. The former are only partly affected by genetics; the latter are almost entirely driven by genetics. With the latter, embryo editing would reduce the risk of disease from one hundred percent to zero. With the former, the situation is not so black and white; the baseline risk is much less than one hundred percent, and embryo editing can at best partially reduce the risk.

With all of these differences, it makes sense to separate coronary artery disease, Alzheimer's disease, and breast cancer from sickle cell disease and cystic fibrosis into two different categories of use of human embryo editing. But where to draw the line is not so clear. Take the example of Huntington's disease. It is similar to sickle cell disease and cystic fibrosis in that if you have the mutation, you will inevitably get the disease. Worse, it is an invariably fatal disease. Embryo editing could reduce the risk of disease from one hundred percent to zero. But unlike sickle cell disease and cystic fibrosis, Huntington's disease only strikes in adulthood, typically between thirty and fifty years of age. It doesn't cause suffering throughout childhood. People who will ultimately develop Huntington's disease have the opportunity to live healthy and productive lives until the disease emerges. So is the rationale for the use of embryo editing to prevent Huntington's disease as strong, or less strong, compared to the rationale to prevent sickle cell disease and cystic fibrosis?

Now consider JK's pursuit of embryo editing of *CCR5*—resulting in the births of Lulu and Nana—to confer resistance to HIV infection. This would seem to be of a piece with the use of embryo editing to reduce the risk of heart disease, Alzheimer's disease, or breast cancer. JK's rationale was that the twins would have been at risk for HIV infection if nothing had been done. With the editing, he substantially reduced their risk (though not to zero, since *CCR5* deletion wouldn't protect against all strains of the virus). But does this argument really hold water? The prevalence of HIV infection in China is less than one tenth of one percent. There's no reason why the twins' risk of HIV infection would have been higher than the risk borne by any of their peers. With editing, the twins' risk was reduced from less than one tenth of one percent to … also less than one tenth of one percent, but still greater than zero. Even in the unlikely circumstance that one of the twins became infected with HIV, with currently available medications there would be little chance of her suffering from AIDS. So did the embryo editing achieve any meaningful change, after all?

The third reason to perform human embryo editing would be enhancement. It is difficult to define exactly what enhancement means. One possible definition: a desirable non-medical trait, that is, one that doesn't directly improve one's health or lifespan. (With the caveat that what is considered desirable is in the eye of the beholder.) Enhancements could range from fairly serious alterations, such as improved intelligence or athletic ability, to what most people would probably consider frivolous changes, such as eye color or hair color.

One problem with this definition is that it can be devilishly difficult—perhaps impossible—to cleanly separate medical traits and non-medical traits. Since shortly after his laboratory and others reported CRISPR-Cas9 gene editing in mammalian cells in 2013, Dr. George Church at Harvard Medical School has included in some of his scientific talks a list of naturally occurring gene mutations that result in desirable traits. The traits include reduced risk of coronary artery disease, Alzheimer's disease, cancer, or diabetes; virus resistance; insensitivity to pain; extra-strong bones; lean muscles; and low body-odor production. Most people would agree that the traits at the beginning of this list can mean life or death, whereas the traits at the end of this list are more cosmetic in nature. But imagine using gene editing to introduce these mutations into embryos for the purpose of introducing these traits. Where to draw the line between medical treatments and enhancements? That is open to debate.

It is a debate that has both moral and economic implications. Talk of editing human embryos for the purpose of enhancement rather than medical therapy has a way of inspiring strong opinions, ranging from accusations of playing God to declarations that it is our responsibility to do everything to improve the human species. There is also the concern that the availability of genetic enhancement will exacerbate already considerable socioeconomic inequities. If it eventually comes to pass that human embryo editing is broadly accepted and available, it is plausible that health insurance plans (whether public or private) will cover it when used in cases of compelling medical need. Prevention of a life-threatening disease is typically cheaper than treating the disease after it has already manifested.

But non-medical enhancements certainly won't be covered. Enhancements will become the province of the wealthy who can afford to pay for them out of pocket. Consider the lengths to which some affluent parents will go for the sake of their children, such as paying to place a child on a years-long waiting list for an elite preschool as soon as the child's been born or, in an extreme example, engaging in illegal activities such as falsifying entrance exam scores and bribing college officials to boost their kid's chance of attending a prestigious university. It's not such a stretch to imagine such parents spending heavily to confer genetic enhancements on their babies before they're born. (Nor is it a stretch to imagine fertility clinics taking advantage of these parents.)

Perhaps it is fortunate, then, that genetic enhancements might not be straightforward to achieve. One complicating factor is that some of the more desirable traits one might wish to instill in one's child, such as enhanced intelligence, are well beyond the reach of gene editing. We are nowhere near an understanding of how genetics influences intelligence, except to say it reflects the interplay of many genes with many non-genetic factors—parenting, peers, access to educational opportunities, nutrition, and exposure to chemicals and toxins, to name a few.

Any single genetic change will at best minimally affect intelligence. (One exception would be the correction of a mutation that causes a disease that substantially impairs cognitive development, but that would be more in the nature of a medical therapy than an enhancement.) It would take the simultaneous modification of numerous genes—probably hundreds— to substantially increase intelligence. With the current state of knowledge, we don't even know with which genes to start. For these same reasons, the well-worn science fiction trope of genetically engineered super-soldiers won't become a reality anytime soon, even if some government were to give its scientists a blank check and full sanction to use gene-editing technology on embryos.

Another complicating factor is the tendency of gene mutations to have a multitude of consequences. A single mutation could have both medically beneficial effects as well as detrimental effects. There is perhaps no better example case study for this phenomenon than *CCR5*, the gene edited in Lulu and Nana. The *CCR5* Δ32 mutation confers resistance to most HIV strains, at least when it is present in two copies. But the same *CCR5* Δ32 mutation also increases vulnerability to other viruses: West Nile virus, tick-borne encephalitis virus, and influenza.

In the months following JK's announcement of the gene-edited twins, it emerged that *CCR5* might be even more complex in its effects on the body than anyone realized. In February 2019, a team of researchers led by Dr. S. Thomas Carmichael at the University of California, Los Angeles, with collaborators at multiple institutions in Israel, reported that stroke patients with at least one copy of the *CCR5* Δ32 mutation showed modestly improved recovery from the stroke, including cognitive function. This was backed up by complementary evidence from mice with stroke or brain injury, in which turning down CCR5 activity also improved recovery and cognitive function. This suggests that Lulu or Nana might have a better outcome if either should ever suffer a stroke—something not intended by JK when he edited the embryos to confer HIV resistance. It would be an unexpected medical benefit.

The researchers also reported something even more provocative: they had preliminary evidence that people with *CCR5* Δ32 mutations achieved a higher level of education. This led to headlines like the one used by Antonio Regalado for his story in *MIT Technology Review*: "China's CRISPR twins might have had their brains inadvertently enhanced." While a lot more evidence will be needed to confirm this assertion, it points to the possibility that the editing of *CCR5* might have crossed over the line between desirable medical traits and unambiguous enhancement—without JK realizing what he was doing.

In June 2019, the potential dangers of making changes in the genome were brought into sharp relief by a report from Drs. Xinzhu Wei and Rasmus Nielsen at the University of California, Berkeley. By studying several hundred thousand people in the United Kingdom, the researchers found that individuals with two copies of the *CCR5 Δ32* mutation had reduced life expectancy. The reason underlying this unsettling observation was unclear. There was speculation that susceptibility to viral infections like flu might account for it. Not surprisingly, the news headlines were rather different than the ones a few months earlier. From Regalado: "'Foolish choice': Rogue Chinese scientist He Jiankui's gene-edited twin babies face risk of premature death."

Even if this observation about reduced lifespan isn't confirmed by future studies, there is an important lesson to be learned about unintended consequences. There are too many unknowns when it comes to genetics. We are just barely starting to understand how single genes affect the body, in good ways and bad ways, and there certainly will be many surprises to come. Rushing ahead, right now, with editing of any gene for any reason other than an extremely compelling medical need seems like folly.

To recap: the three use cases for human embryo editing are (1) to eliminate a grievous genetic disease that otherwise would be certain to happen, (2) to significantly reduce the risk of a disease occurring during the lifetime, and (3) enhancement. As we have seen, the lines between these use cases can be quite blurry. Any attempts to legislate or regulate editing of embryos using these strict definitions—for example, permitting the first category but banning the second and third categories—will be fraught with challenges.

Still, it's instructive to feel out what members of the general public think about gene-edited babies. JK's actions did little to place human embryo editing in a positive light. But it seems that the general condemnation that greeted JK's announcement of Lulu and Nana had more to do with his sloppy science, the lack of a medical need, his secrecy, and his profound ethical breaches, rather than the existence of gene-edited babies per se. Certainly nobody has been questioning Lulu's and Nana's standing as human beings and citizens.

After the first report of gene editing in (non-viable) human embryos by a team of Chinese researchers in 2015, various groups commissioned polls of the general public about the prospect of gene-edited babies. One early poll in the United States by the Pew Research Center in 2016 asked, "If you had a baby, do you think this gene-editing—giving a much reduced risk of serious diseases and conditions over his or her lifetime—is something that you, personally, would want for your baby or not something you would want for your baby?" Opinions were evenly split, with forty-eight percent responding that they would "definitely" or "probably want this for their baby." There was a similar divergence of opinions for the somewhat different question, "If this gene-editing becomes available giving healthy babies a much reduced risk of serious diseases and conditions, do you think there would be …," thirty-six percent completed the sentence with "more benefits for society than downsides," thirty-three percent with "about equal benefits and downsides for society," and twenty-eight percent with "more downsides for society than benefits." In this poll, respondents who were familiar with gene editing were more likely to want it for their babies, and those who felt religion was important to them were less likely to want gene editing for their babies.

Another poll in the United States performed in 2016, this one by *STAT* and Harvard T.H. Chan School of Public Health, found a more pessimistic outlook. When asked, "Do you think that changing the genes of unborn babies to reduce their risk of developing certain serious diseases should be legal or should be illegal?," only twenty-six percent felt it should be legal. When asked, "Do you think that changing the genes of unborn babies to improve their intelligence or physical characteristics should be legal or should be illegal?," even fewer felt it should be legal, just eleven percent. One curious finding: when asked, "For decisions on whether or not to allow changing the genes of unborn babies to improve their healthy, physical traits, or intelligence, do you think we should leave it up to ...," the majority, fifty-three percent, agreed with "scientists, physicians, and other technological experts." Only nine percent agreed with "government officials and policy makers." Of course, it is the latter group of people who ultimately decide what is legal and what is illegal.

Still, I was encouraged by the relatively high level of trust the public seems to have in scientists and physicians to weigh in on thorny issues like human embryo editing. This inspired me to perform a poll of my own with attendees at a large scientific conference. I explored the differences between the three use cases. When I asked, "Do you think it would be acceptable for parents to use human germline genome editing to have a healthy biological child when there is no other means to do so?," sixty-one percent said yes and twenty-eight percent said no (the others being undecided). When I changed the question, "... to reduce the risk of their child having a serious medical condition (for example, premature coronary heart disease or Alzheimer's disease)?," there was slightly less support, with forty-five percent saying yes, and forty percent saying no. With the final question, "... to increase the odds of their child having a desired trait (for example, athletic ability)?," support plummeted to just two percent saying yes, and ninety-five percent saying no.

The overwhelmingly negative news stories about JK's actions with respect to Lulu and Nana don't seem to have undermined support for human embryo editing among the U.S. public. If anything, support appears to have increased over the past few years. In an Associated Press–NORC Center for Public Affairs Research poll taken a few weeks after JK's announcement, about seventy percent of respondents favored medical uses of embryo editing, whether it involved "preventing an incurable or fatal disease that a child would inherit, such as cystic fibrosis or Huntington's," "reducing the risk of diseases, such as cancer, that might develop later in life," or "preventing a non-fatal condition that a child would inherit, such as blindness." Only about ten percent of respondents favored enhancements, namely "altering capabilities such as intelligence or athletic ability" or "altering physical characteristics such as eye color or height."

These various polls suggest that it will be very difficult to achieve a consensus on the broad use of gene editing in human embryos. But it does seem there could eventually be strong majorities for or against specific use cases. There's certainly much more sympathy for parents who would be unable to have healthy biological children without gene editing than for parents who would seek to use gene editing to make their child better than everyone else's.

Even if there turns out to be broad public support to proceed with human embryo editing, JK's clinical trial demonstrated that gene-editing technology is nowhere near ready for use in embryos. The undesirable consequences of gene editing that emerged in JK's work—mosaicism and off-target effects—aren't close to being solved. Indeed, it's not clear that they can be solved in embryos.

Why is this? Recall that JK's team injected CRISPR-Cas9 directly into single-cell zygotes and grew them into blastocysts. They then carried out pre-implantation genetic diagnosis—out of the two to three hundred cells in the embryo, taking three to five cells for DNA analysis. These few cells have to be destroyed in order to get at the DNA and perform sequencing. The usefulness of the analysis is entirely predicated on the assumption that these few cells have exactly the same genomes, including any on-target and off-target edits, as the remainder of the embryo. With Lulu's and Nana's embryos, with their known mosaicism, that assumption was unequivocally a bad one. JK couldn't be sure what was going on in the remainder of each embryo, the cells that ended up becoming the body of one of the twins.

And there is no technique that would have allowed him to directly analyze the DNA in the future body of the child before establishing the pregnancy.

For anyone attempting to perform human embryo editing in the future, the same problem will be there. Because gene editing has the potential to cause different edits in different cells in the embryo, what's happening in all of the cells of the embryo besides the few cells sacrificed for DNA analysis is unknowable. Which means that establishing a pregnancy with an edited embryo will always be a roll of the dice. It's possible that amniocentesis—the process of using a needle inserted into the uterus and amniotic sac to collect cells shed into the fluid surrounding the fetus during pregnancy—could provide an early look at what's in the DNA of the future child. But the cells shed from the fetus might not be same as all of the other cells in the fetus. It's possible that if the shed cells looked correct, there might still be undetected mosaicism and off-target mutations somewhere in the body of the fetus. If amniocentesis did reveal problems with the fetus, the choice would be to allow the baby to come to term and hope for the best or to undergo an elective abortion. It's not a choice that a parent ever wants to face.

There's actually a solution to this problem, but it would involve gene editing before the embryo even exists. The editing would take place in cells that are subsequently used to make embryos. One possibility would be to make edits directly in sperm cells or egg cells (together known as gametes). A gene-editing tool like CRISPR-Cas9 would be injected directly into the gametes or introduced into the gametes another way, perhaps through the use of chemicals or an electrical charge to temporarily open up holes in the surfaces of the cells. The gametes would be maintained long enough to allow CRISPR-Cas9 to make the desired edits and then dissipate. Then the edited gametes would be used to make single-cell zygotes by in vitro fertilization. This wouldn't be embryo editing, per se, but it would enable transmission of edited genes to offspring. In scientific parlance, this would be germline gene editing. (This is in contrast to somatic gene editing, which describes editing within a person's body that wouldn't be passed to the next generation.)

The advantage of gamete editing over doing the editing in the zygote is that the editing would be guaranteed to be finished well before the zygote is made. The zygote would then divide into the numerous cells of the embryo—and every cell would carry the same edits. At the blastocyst stage, each embryo would undergo pre-implantation genetic diagnosis. The assumption that the analyzed three to five cells would match the other two to three hundred cells of the blastocyst would be valid, at least with respect to the edits. So mosaicism of the edits wouldn't be a concern. Any embryos found to have the desired on-target edits, and to not have any off-target edits, could then be used to establish a pregnancy.

Yet the gene editing need not occur directly in the gametes. It could occur even earlier, in the cells from which gametes arise. In the testicles, spermatogonial stem cells are the precursor cells that give rise to all of the sperm. Being stem cells, theoretically they can divide and grow indefinitely and provide an everlasting source of sperm. Although methods to grow human spermatogonial stem cells outside of the body, in the laboratory, have yet to be perfected, it's become quite routine with mouse spermatogonial stem cells. In fact, it's possible to transplant donor spermatogonial stem cells into the testicles of infertile mice and restore their fertility—a technique that might one day enable infertile men to sire children.

In 2014, a group of Chinese researchers led by Dr. Jinsong Li at the Shanghai Institutes for Biological Sciences reported the first use of CRISPR-Cas9 in spermatogonial stem cells. In their study, they isolated spermatogonial stem cells from mice with cataracts resulting from two mutant copies of the *Crygc* gene. They grew these cells in dishes in the laboratory, treated them with CRISPR-Cas9, and identified single cells in which the mutations had been corrected. The researchers then performed genome sequencing to ensure the cells didn't have any off-target mutations. Finally, they grew the corrected cells into large numbers and transplanted them into the testicles of infertile male mice. Now back in their native environment, the edited spermatogonial stem cells produced mature sperm, which were then used to generate offspring mice. The young mice, as hoped, had the corrected *Crygc* gene and were free of cataracts.

This work didn't attract much attention when it was published, but it might hold the key to someday allowing parents to safely use germline gene editing to spare their children from disease, avoiding the problems of embryo editing.

There's an even more exotic way in which one might indirectly introduce edits into the germline. One could take a blood sample or skin sample from a prospective parent and reprogram the cells into induced pluripotent stem cells. Recall that these cells have the unusual capacity to be turned into any of the body's cell types. Theoretically, it should be possible to create egg cells or sperm cells from any person's induced pluripotent stem cells. In October 2018, just one month before JK's announcement of the gene-edited twins, a team of Japanese researchers led by Dr. Mitinori Saitou at Kyoto University made headlines by publishing a study in which they successfully coaxed human induced pluripotent stem cells into becoming egg-like cells. The process involved a number of steps, turning the cells from one type into another type into another and then another. The key step was incubating the human cells in tiny artificial ovaries the researchers had created from mouse cells especially for that purpose.

The final eggs didn't seem to be mature enough to be viable. Certainly the researchers had no intention of testing these human eggs by trying to fertilize them and establish a pregnancy. But two years earlier, the same team had shown they could make mature eggs from mouse stem cells and use the eggs to produce live, healthy offspring. And several years before that, the team had shown they could do the same with sperm made from mouse stem cells. So the new work with human cells opened the door to the possibility of creating eggs or sperm on demand, even from people who otherwise wouldn't be able to produce viable gametes because of age or infertility. The potential ethical stickiness was pointed out by Dr. Ronald Green, a bioethicist at Dartmouth College, to *NPR*: "A woman might want to have George Clooney's baby. And his hairdresser could start selling his hair follicles online. So we suddenly could see many, many progeny of George Clooney without his consent."

One cardinal advantage of induced pluripotent stem cells is that they're highly amenable to gene editing, with multiple edits being quite feasible. Not too far in the future, there might be no technical bar to the following scenario. A person visits a clinic to have induced pluripotent stem cells made. Upon request, the clinic edits out a disease-causing mutation, or edits in a disease-protecting alteration, or edits in an enhancement—or all of the above. Then the clinic performs intensive quality control with genome sequencing and other methods to make sure the stem cells have the desired edits and no undesired edits. The cells are turned into sperm or eggs, which are then used for in vitro fertilization. The resulting embryos are screened again with pre-implantation genetic diagnosis to make sure they have only the desired edits. On toward pregnancy, and finally the birth of the much-anticipated child.

This scenario reads so much like science fiction that no existing laws or regulations really address it. The direct editing of embryos is problematic in many countries. In the United States, a provision of federal law currently makes it prohibited to proceed with medical applications "in which a human embryo is intentionally created or modified to include a heritable genetic modification." (Though it is worth noting that this particular provision came close to being stripped from the law by the U.S. Congress in 2019.) But what if the editing were to occur in cells that aren't typically regarded as the germline, that is, not embryos and not gametes?

Making induced pluripotent stem cells is being done for tens of thousands of people. Editing of stem cells in a dish has become routine. Turning stem cells into gametes in a dish isn't intrinsically all that different from turning them into heart muscle cells, or liver cells, or brain cells, which is happening in many laboratories around the world. In vitro fertilization for reproductive purposes is a well-accepted and commonly performed medical procedure, resulting in millions of babies. The only step that might be tricky is using stem cell-derived gametes for in vitro fertilization, regardless of whether or not the stem cells had been edited. If governments decide this step is problematic, they will have to craft new laws and regulations to prevent it.

How soon can we expect the newest members of the CRISPR generation to be born, to join Lulu and Nana? Is there anything the international biomedical community can do to prevent or even just delay more births? A review of the events of the past few years don't provide much reason for optimism for those opposed to human embryo editing.

Dr. Jennifer Doudna at the University of California, Berkeley, often tells a story of a nightmare in which Adolf Hitler asked her about CRISPR technology and how it could be used. She woke up in a cold sweat, horrified about what somebody with Hitler's eugenics ideology might try to do with gene editing. In early 2015, having caught wind that Chinese scientists were experimenting with gene editing in human embryos, Doudna organized a group of biologists and ethicists who met in Napa, California, to discuss the scientific, medical, legal, and ethical implications of gene-editing technology. They subsequently published a perspective piece in the journal *Science* that was widely interpreted as a call for a worldwide moratorium on human embryo editing. At around the same time, another group writing in the journal *Nature* explicitly called for "a voluntary moratorium in the scientific community."

One month later came the publication of the first paper reporting gene editing in human embryos. This event provided the impetus for the convening of the International Summit on Human Gene Editing in Washington, DC, in December 2015, hosted by the U.S. National Academy of Sciences, U.S. National Academy of Medicine, Chinese Academy of Sciences, and the Royal Society of London. After three days of talks by scientists, ethicists, policymakers, patient advocates, and other stakeholders, the organizing committee released a summary statement outlining the benefits and risks of human gene editing. Although the statement didn't include the word "moratorium," it did make the following appeal:

> "It would be irresponsible to proceed with any clinical use of germline editing unless and until (i) the relevant safety and efficacy issues have been resolved, based on appropriate understanding and balancing of risks, potential benefits, and alternatives, and (ii) there is broad societal consensus about the appropriateness of the proposed application. Moreover, any clinical use should proceed only under appropriate regulatory oversight. At present, these criteria have not been met for any proposed clinical use: the safety issues have not yet been adequately explored; the cases of most compelling benefit are limited; and many nations have legislative or regulatory bans on germline modification. However, as scientific knowledge advances and societal views evolve, the clinical use of germline editing should be revisited on a regular basis."

JK was paying attention. He apparently interpreted the statement as a yellow light rather than a red light. In his mind, he was free to move ahead once he fulfilled the conditions laid out by the committee. After a couple of years of work, he could show that he had adequately addressed condition (i) through his laboratory's research on mouse, monkey, and human embryos. He felt that his application of gene-editing technology was effective and safe enough to proceed with a clinical trial.

To satisfy condition (ii), JK simply looked to the surveys taken in the United States and elsewhere suggesting that there was substantial support among the general public for human embryo editing in cases of medical need. In his single scientific presentation after announcing the births of Lulu and Nana, he spoke to this issue. "My original plan, original thinking was based on the survey of the United States or the U.S. or the British ethics statement or the Chinese study that gave us the signal that the majority of the public is supporting using the human genome editing for treating, including HIV prevention."

Finally, JK could make the claim that he was proceeding "under appropriate regulatory oversight." The laws and regulations in China were ambiguous when it came to human embryo editing, and he was able to show off a signed approval document from a hospital's research ethics committee.

One wonders whether JK wouldn't have proceeded with his clinical trial if the statement released at the end of the International Summit on Human Gene Editing had been more firmly opposed to human embryo editing or had come out more explicitly in favor of a moratorium. Or whether JK's desire to make history by becoming the first to create gene-edited babies was so overwhelming that he would have gone ahead anyway, and then come up with other excuses to retrospectively justify his actions. In 2017, a writing group convened by the U.S. National Academies as a follow-up to the International Summit published a lengthy report that laid out somewhat stricter criteria that should be fulfilled before a clinical trial of human embryo editing could be permitted. It does not appear to have deterred JK in any way.

At the end of the International Summit, it was understood that discussions would be ongoing, and that there would be a need for future meetings. The groundwork was laid for a Second International Summit on Human Genome Editing, which ultimately would take place in Hong Kong in November 2018, three years after the first Summit and involving many of the same organizers. And in an unfortunate coincidence of timing, the agenda of the Second International Summit would be hijacked by JK's public announcement of the gene-edited twins and his presentation at the Summit.

Some observers were appalled that the Summit organizers had given JK a prominent forum in which to present his work to a global audience. Even more were disappointed at the statement from the organizers at the end of the meeting. Concerning human germline editing: "The variability of effects produced by genetic changes makes it difficult to conduct a thorough evaluation of benefits and risks. Nevertheless, germline genome editing could become acceptable in the future if these risks are addressed and if a number of additional criteria are met. These criteria include strict independent oversight, a compelling medical need, an absence of reasonable alternatives, a plan for long-term follow-up, and attention to societal effects. Even so, public acceptability will likely vary among jurisdictions, leading to differing policy responses."

Although the statement did make note of JK's announcement, there was a widespread perception that the organizers didn't do enough to try to deter scientists from following in JK's footsteps. The yellow light was still a yellow light, not a red light. If anything, the new statement was weaker than the one from the first Summit three years earlier. It no longer talked about anyone proceeding with germline editing being "irresponsible" or mentioned the need for a "broad societal consensus." It certainly didn't come anywhere close to calling for an immediate moratorium. This perception was only amplified by a comment from Dr. George Daley of Harvard Medical School, one of the conference organizers: "The fact that the first instance of human germline editing came forward as a misstep should not let us stick our neck in the sand."

Nonetheless, JK's announcement did spur some action. The World Health Organization convened an Advisory Committee on Developing Global Standards for Governance and Oversight of Human Genome Editing. The Advisory Committee was "tasked to advise and make recommendations on appropriate institutional, national, regional, and global governance mechanisms for human genome editing." The U.S. National Academy of Medicine, U.S. National Academy of Sciences, and Royal Society of London—the same groups involved with the two Summits—

announced an International Commission on the Clinical Use of Human Germline Genome Editing. Its purpose would be to create a framework to "identify a number of scientific, medical, and ethical requirements that should be considered, and could inform the development of a potential pathway from research to clinical use—if society concludes that heritable human genome editing applications are acceptable."

In its first meeting in March 2019, the World Health Organization Advisory Committee recommended the creation of a global registry for all human gene-editing research. The idea was that all researchers in the field would register their work and receive registration numbers. Ideally, funding organizations, whether governments or private funders, would require their funding recipients to participate in the registry, and scientific journals would only publish human gene-editing research if there was a registration number. Scientists who wished to receive funding and publish their work would have a strong incentive to cooperate.

Still, the registry would be voluntary. It's not clear that its existence would have deterred JK from proceeding with his clinical trial. He was, after all, a self-funded researcher who announced Lulu and Nana to the world via YouTube and press outreach rather than a scientific publication. And that highlights the major limitation of the two international committees' work. Having no force of law to back up their recommendations, the committees will function in an advisory role only. It's ultimately up to governments to decide whether to heed the recommendations and incorporate them into their laws.

The early indications are that efforts by these international committees to prevent the births of more gene-edited babies, before safety and efficacy and compelling medical need are established to everybody's satisfaction, might be ineffectual. In June 2019, a Russian scientist, Dr. Denis Rebrikov at the Kulakov National Medical Research Center of Obstetrics, Gynecology and Perinatology in Moscow, made headlines by announcing his intention to proceed with the editing of human embryos in order to make gene-edited babies.

Rebrikov first shared the details in a news story in *Nature*. His plans came across as a sorry rehash of JK's discredited clinical trial. He intended to go after the same gene, *CCR5*, for the same reason, to confer HIV resistance. He claimed that his justification was stronger than JK's. Instead of targeting HIV-positive fathers, he would target HIV-positive mothers who had responded poorly to antiviral therapy and were more likely to pass HIV to their infants. In an interview with *Science*, he conceded there were only about thirty such women in Russia. If he couldn't find any willing volunteers, he would then try parents who both had a recessive genetic condition like "dwarfism, deafness, or blindness."

Rebrikov claimed to have a "unique" gene-editing system that was superior to JK's. It would introduce precise copies of the *CCR5 Δ32* mutation and eliminate off-target mutations. He pointed to a paper published in the local journal *Bulletin of the RSMU*, of which he just so happened to be editor-in-chief, as evidence of his prowess. But a quick read of the paper reveals amateurish work that doesn't come close to the level of a genuine gene-editing expert; it even falls short of the shoddy standards set by JK in his clinical trial.

If there's one positive thing to be said of Rebrikov, it's that unlike JK, he couldn't be faulted for being secretive about his plans. (Though some commentators wondered if Rebrikov had no serious intention of creating gene-edited babies but was simply making a cynical play for publicity—in which case, mission accomplished.) Rebrikov told *Nature* that he would seek approvals from three Russian government agencies, including the health ministry, before proceeding. With those approvals in hand, he would go forward with the editing if he was convinced of the safety of the procedure. "I think I'm crazy enough to do it."

When asked by *Science* what he thought of the use of human embryo editing for enhancement, Rebrikov was unsubtle in his response. "It will be the next step. But in twenty to thirty years. Now, I'm opposed to it. In 2040, I will support it. I'm not against the idea itself. And these people who are opposed want to have all these things in their children but only by 'divine providence,' not by science. They are liars or stupid." And when it was pointed out to him that there were two international committees that would be discussing the best path forward to regulate embryo editing: "I don't think it's possible to restrict some experiments worldwide … We can't stop progress with words on paper." When asked by *STAT* what they could do to prevent Rebrikov from going forward, both Dr. Margaret Hamburg, co-chair of the World Health Organization's Advisory Committee, and Dr. Victor Dzau, president of the U.S. National Academy of Medicine and co-chair of the oversight board of the International Commission, conceded that there was little they could do to stop him.

So things stand in the autumn of 2019. Lulu and Nana are the first recognized members of the CRISPR generation. Who will be the next one? Will it be a baby born from the second pregnancy from JK's clinical trial? Will it be a baby born in Russia as a result of Rebrikov's efforts? Will it be a baby born from a pregnancy that's already underway, for now hidden from the world by some unnamed scientist or physician? Will we even find out about it when it happens?

Lulu and Nana were born forty years after Louise Brown, the first test tube baby from in vitro fertilization. The circumstances of Brown's birth were controversial at the time. So it's remarkable that millions of babies are now being born from in vitro fertilization. It's become an accepted part of everyday life.

Will the same be true of gene-edited babies? Will the CRISPR generation in forty years be much larger than anyone dares to imagine now?